Effective Birth Preparation
YOUR PRACTICAL GUIDE TO A BETTER BIRTH

by
Maggie Howell

Founder and Director of Natal Hypnotherapy

Published by
Intuition UN Ltd

2009

Effective Birth Preparation
Your practical guide to a better birth

Published by Intuition UN Ltd
        Unit 2
        Riverside business park
        Farnham
        Surrey
        GU9 7SS
        Tel +44 01252 716859

ISBN 978-1-905220-59-5
EAN 9781905220595

To my wonderful husband, who has supported me, guided me, uplifted me and inspired me through my amazing journey as a mother, a therapist and a writer.

Plus a special thank you to all the women and men who have volunteered to share their birth stories in this book. All of them used the Natal Hypnotherapy techniques, either by listening to the tracks or attending the course.

Reviews of The Effective Birth Preparation - Your practical guide to a better birth

Sheila Kitzinger, MBE – Author, honorary professor teaching an MA in midwifery, anthropologist, campaigner for natural birth

"Here is a fascinating and impressive book that empowers a woman to prepare for birth by drawing on her own inner resources – she doesn't have to depend on others to discipline and train her, but through insight and understanding, and using skills of relaxation, rhythmic breathing, and the art of creative imagination, she can focus on the birth energy released in her body.

She learns to manage pain and face the challenge of labour, whether it is fast or slow, and she is under her own control, nobody else's.

The material is well researched and vividly presented, and any woman who studies and rehearses the author's practical suggestions helps herself towards a positive – even exultant – birth experience."

Khim Lee – Midwife, antenatal teacher, mother

"How empowering and rewarding it is for me, as a midwife, to see how effective the techniques in this book are. They have made a tremendous contribution to women, enabling them to have better birth experiences.

Midwifery is becoming too medicalised and often contradicts what NICE Guidelines recommend in Normalising Maternity care. I feel that all midwives should really be trained in Natal Hypnotherapy, as the techniques are effective, simple tools which will also help make midwives better and more sensitive and caring, thus helping women have calmer birth experiences."

Ellie Hughes – Editor, *Pregnancy & Birth* magazine, mother of two

"Whatever your views on the kind of birth you think you would like, you will find plenty here to help you work with your body, and feel confident and in control during this life-changing, life-giving event. A huge help in combating the fears many women will feel as they approach labour."

Shona Kitchener – Mother, champion of natural parenting, animal behavioural scientist

"This book is a pocket-sized course & therapy session in one. I found reading the book cleansing, inspiring, encouraging and empowering. It has left me filled with a deep sense of power and pride when reflecting on the birth of my daughter and with a sense of urgency when considering doing it all again!

The most beautiful part for me was that, rather than talking about replacing negative images and thoughts with positive ones (a near-impossible task for most mums of my generation, as there are so few to replace them with!), this book provides what all the others have missed by offering wonderful stories and experiences, as told by mothers who have used Natal Hypnotherapy. Each story is told with perfect timing in the book, and many are so memorable and moving that I found that they went straight into my subconscious, as if to cleanse the old ones away. It is written so naturally and from the heart that everything sounds instantly familiar and right.

This book is a life-changing read and should be on every pregnant mum's essential-purchases list!"

Julie Green – Midwifery lecturer; Supervisor of Midwives – LSA Midwife; Director – Birth and Beyond Consultancy Ltd.

"Maggie describes the tools required for instinctive birthing so well – this book will help women to reduce any fear they may have before the phenomenal, life-changing event of birth. The non-technical explanations and use of women's stories reflect the body's natural ability to give birth so positively, giving control back to the woman herself – excellent."

Dot Parry – Midwife, NCT teacher, mother

"This modern-day manual is packed with old-fashioned wisdom and common-sense techniques to help twenty-first-century women give birth confidently, safely and   peacefully."

Emma Rhodes – Natal Hypnotherapy mother

"Reading this book is like having an enormous weight lifted. It's so refreshing, encouraging and full of good sense, convincing you that not only is a calm, relaxed, positive birth experience entirely possible – it should be expected!"

Danielle Diosi – NCT teacher, twins' antenatal teacher, mother to twins

"The thing that stuck out for me when reading this wonderful book was how much sense it made. It makes everything very clear and really emphasises the point that birth is not rocket science – it is just a normal physiological process. A definite must for any pregnant woman's reading list."

Caroline Baddiley – Independent midwife

"How wonderfully refreshing to have a birth-preparation book that focuses on feelings and emotions rather than on the technicalities of birth.

A complete how-to-deal-with-fear toolkit for all pregnant women."

Michel Odent MD – Author, surgeon, obstetrician, founder of the Primal Health Research Centre, present at over 15,000 births

"The book by Maggie Howell is much more than a practical guide for birth preparation. It is a book about human nature. It includes several dominant themes. One of them is the negative effect, in certain situations, of the knowledge that human adults have acquired, compared in particular with the knowledge transmitted from generation to generation among non-human animals.

Obviously, Maggie has digested the contents of the first pages of the bestseller written several thousand years ago. She has been able to interpret 'the sin of consuming the fruit of the tree of knowledge', and she has noticed the significant association, in the first pages of this famous ancient book, between knowing too much and being condemned to have difficult birth.

In modern scientific language we can explain this association by introducing the concept of neocortical inhibition, and by claiming that **the huge development of the neocortex – the brain of the intellect – is the main reason for difficult births in our species.** *The solution to cope with this human handicap is to put the neocortex at rest.*

This is why 'Natal Hypnotherapy' can be presented as a set of tools to overcome powerful neocortical inhibitions and the effects of thousands of years of cultural conditioning."

Contents

Preface

"If you have knowledge, let others light their candles in it" – Margaret Fuller

The concepts and techniques explained in this book, have grown and developed organically in the UK since 2000. They were born out of the philosophy that childbirth is a normal, natural part of life and that we as humans are essentially mammals and so have the innate knowledge to birth our babies.

During the pregnancy of my first son, I became acutely aware of how frightened most women were about giving birth, and felt sad and bemused that birth had become viewed as an ordeal, a painful, frightening experience that you had to endure. I was also astonished at the number of medical interventions required by so many women and surprised at how few positive stories I heard about giving birth.

When I first heard about the use of hypnosis for childbirth, I was not totally convinced and still wondered how using the power of your mind could really make any difference to the physical act of childbirth. Even though I strongly believed that my body would know what to do, and possibly because my mother had had her labour induced for my birth, I still subconsciously feared that the birth would be incredibly painful. However, the more I practised the hypnosis and relaxation, the more confident and calm I felt. I had chosen to have a home birth, and so felt very comfortable and at ease with my surroundings, which I knew would make a big difference.

On the day that I went into labour, I felt calm and relaxed at all times. I had a long labour but one which was steady, unrushed, quiet and calm. I was not really aware at the time that the hypnosis was "working" – it was really in hindsight that I realised how much of what I had practised and rehearsed seemed to come true.

So was it painful? At times, yes, but never to the point where I felt out of control or unable to deal with it. I never once felt fear of the process itself and so was able to go with each sensation, accepting each one as part of my birth experience.

My first experience of birth was calm, empowering, intense, animalistic, powerful and long. Did I feel out of control? No. Did I need any pain relief? No. Did I want to do it all over again? Absolutely!

A grand adventure is about to begin – Winnie the Pooh

It was a true passage to womanhood. I felt my body move and open in ways that I had never experienced before; I felt an intensity and power that only a birthing woman can feel; I felt the limits of my body's amazing abilities go to the extreme; I felt lost in a dreamy world of intense, powerful sensations which I had no control over.

I needed no one, I needed nothing, I had handed control over to my body – all I had was trust, instinct and an incredible source of energy. My body was in its element, and I was at my most supreme – it was the accumulation of every day since my birth. I was doing what my body was put on this planet to do – I was bringing new life into this world, and I loved it!

And that is the essence of Natal Hypnotherapy. It is about rekindling that awesome power within women. It is about rebuilding the trust a woman feels about her own body. It is about empowering her to follow her instincts.

The modern world's approach to birth has stripped away so many of these things. Women have lost that trust, that confidence, the sense of power and awe in their own ability. It has been replaced by fear, anxiety, and subservience to the medical world. A new belief has arisen: that a woman needs machines, instruments, tests and other experts to "deliver" her baby.

Natal Hypnotherapy is gradually helping more and more women to move beyond this and back to the way nature intended. Regardless of a woman's birth choices, Natal Hypnotherapy is there to help her feel more confident, more empowered, more in control – to help her tune into her instincts and to feel once again that sense of trust in her body's ability to birth her baby.

Women and their partners come to us to be helped on their journey. They know where they are starting from and where they want to get to. They know the road that they need to take, but they are not yet sure of exactly what they will see on that road or where, and when, the bends will come. There might be some uphill bits and there will probably be some downhill bits. They may even find they get caught in traffic or road works which block them. But, whatever obstacle they meet, our aim is to help them smooth out their journey so that they keep their destination in mind and so that, with persistence and determination, they get there. The journey will take a woman right back to her core – back to where we all started. To a time and place where she can, and will, have rekindled that complete trust and confidence in her body's inherent ability to birth her baby.

A great joy is coming – Author unknown

Many women ask, "Can giving birth be painless?"

Yes, it is possible. However, Natal Hypnotherapy is not about encouraging, endorsing or in any way promising a painless birth. It is about teaching you the tools and techniques to help you overcome fear, be in control, and reduce pain. It teaches you to understand and trust your body, so you hand "control" over from your conscious, intellectual mind to your birthing mind and body.

Natal Hypnotherapy will help you to have a birth which is instinctive, manageable and in some cases even pain free. As with anything, though, this will only be achievable if you can truly trust in your body, believe it is possible, prepare well and practise, practise, practise.

Natal Hypnotherapy is essentially about helping you to be effectively **prepared** for birth, and NOT scared of birth.

As this book goes to print, I am excitedly awaiting the birth of our fifth child. I am loving the anticipation of bringing another wonderful little person into the world and once again relishing the changes in my body and the wonderful excitement of the forthcoming birth.

So, my message to you is: enjoy this book, allow yourself to truly trust your instincts, relish your pregnancy and accept all the emotions you will face.

You may then be surprised how much more you look forward to the birth.

Maggie Howell d.hyp, c.hyp, UK HypReg, NCH, BA Hons.
Founder of Natal Hypnotherapy

Everything grows rounder and wider and weirder, and I sit here in the middle of it all and wonder who in the world you will turn out to be – Carrie Fisher

Before you were conceived I wanted you
Before you were born I loved you
Before you were here an hour I would die for you
This is the miracle of Mother's Love.

Maureen Hawkins

A story

Imagine you are a young woman who has lived her whole life in a remote, tribal community and you are pregnant for the first time. You have grown up in an extended family and have been around women who were pregnant, have given birth and brought up children for as long as you can remember. Your older sister, your cousin and your best friend are also pregnant. Because you live closely together, you have always had your period around the same time and have spent many wonderful days together in a separate area, away from the men, during your menstruation. You are comfortable and at ease with your body and all your body's functions – why shouldn't you be? As a young woman in a small rural community, you have squatted down to take a pee while chatting with your friends, you have bathed naked in the nearby river, and you have made love to your husband within earshot of sleeping relatives.

And you have watched and helped as other women have gone into labour and given birth. You have taken part in wonderful rituals of singing, dancing, and chanting to help the mother flow through the birth. You have been part of the group that brings special gifts and celebration food after the baby has been born. You have combed her hair, oiled her skin and fanned her when she got hot. You have watched her suckling her child; you have watched as she has picked up on her baby's needs; you have noticed how her baby wriggles just before needing a wee; you have watched as she has slept peacefully with her baby in the crook of her arm. When she was ready, you have seen her pop her baby in a simple cloth sling and once again freely go about her daily routine.

For centuries, your people have celebrated birth, and now it is your turn. During your pregnancy, you have been given the best food; you have been massaged and have been the focus of many storytellers. Yet you still work hard, cook food, carry wood and collect water. Your body is strong, fit and healthy. And now you are excited and looking forward to all the caring and attention that comes with having a baby. You are looking forward to going through a rite of passage, another journey to becoming a mother.

And at the same time you know that the birth can take several hours; you know that it is harder work than walking for hours to find firewood; you know that your body will release water and blood. You accept that your stomach will go hard and soft, and that your muscles will ache and burn; you know that your genitals will open and give way for your baby to be born. You know that you may growl and moan like an animal. You will remember the many other births you have seen, remembering how calm and tranquil the mother was, knowing that, even though her body was working hard, she seemed to be in a different place in her mind.

You also know that you will have the love and support of the women you have grown up with around you. You know that they will help you when you feel tired, that they will use chanting and dance to help your body and your baby, that they will massage you and hold you in their arms. You feel safe, warm and connected to those that love you and support you. Everything will be taken care of – you know that there is nothing you need to do, other than to let your body give birth. You know that you can freely surrender to the power and force in your body, which will bring your baby into the world, just as you have seen so many times before.

Introduction

Now take a moment to come back to your reality. I do not know anything about you, the society or culture in which you live, or how you feel about birth; however, I imagine that your feelings about the forthcoming birth will probably differ from this young woman's.

I do not need to tell you that in our so-called modern world, being pregnant and giving birth is far removed from the life and beliefs of this woman. She has many feelings and views of birth, but the one emotion which is not present is fear. She has no need to be frightened. Birth is part of life. Death is part of life. Everyone is born and everyone dies. Everyone eats and everyone goes to the toilet. She does not marvel at her body and she does not fear it – she does not need to. She has a completely natural and in-built trust and belief that her body will do what it needs to in order to digest food, to breathe air, to give birth.

She does not understand how her body gives birth; she has not learnt about the mechanics of birth; she has not learnt about all the things that can go wrong. Why should she? She has the wisdom and experience of the other women round her to help her if need be, women who have seen all kinds of births and who have remedies to help even the hardest births. She knows that if the baby is long in coming, the women will suggest different ways to stand, different ways to move, and different ways to massage her body to help the baby into the best position for birth. She has not been to classes or read books or spent hours on the Internet or watched Discovery Health! She has gathered all the learning she needs from being a part of other women's experiences.

Yes, birth is a part of life, but it is also a wonderful time of celebration, a celebration of life and birth: birth of a mother, birth of a father, and birth of a new baby. A time when she is the focus of attention, when she is nurtured and cared for – a time to look forward to and a time to enjoy.

In our world, we cannot miraculously recreate the small communal environment where it is accepted and encouraged to participate in other women's births. We cannot conjure up extended families. Many of us cannot give birth surrounded by familiar faces in a familiar setting.

Life is magic; the way nature works seems to be quite magical – Jonas Salk

But what is in every woman's power is the ability to reconnect with her body's ability to give birth. You can change your beliefs about birth and you can overcome any fears so that you are more freely able to trust in your body and to hand over control to your body's instinctive functions and processes.

You can also share your positive experiences with other women and so encourage and teach them that birth can be a positive and empowering experience. The more women can share positive stories about birth, the less other women will see birth as something to be frightened of.

Whatever your experiences are – how your mother gave birth to you, what your fears and concerns are, where you plan to give birth – this book will help you prepare positively for the forthcoming birth. By understanding the impact that your thoughts and fears can have on your experiences, specifically on your birth experience, and by learning how to clear the path of obstacles and hurdles, you will be freeing yourself, predominantly your thoughts, so that, when the time comes, your mind will no longer interfere with the already installed bodily functions of giving birth.

Will this book tell you how to give birth?

No.

Unlike many other approaches to birth preparation, this book does not need to tell you how to give birth – there is no need to, as every cell and muscle in your body already knows how to do that. Birth is an involuntary process – just like your digestive system or your blood system. This book will not give you graphic explanations of what happens in each phase of birth. And it will most definitely not tell you about all the things that can go wrong and what to do in each situation – there are plenty of other books that cover that subject!

Will it tell you how to have a pain-free birth?

No.

It is important to remember that nothing worth having in life is completely pain free: relationships, achievements, being a parent, overcoming challenges – these are not pain free. Pain is an integral and important part of life – it can focus the mind, teach you things, make

> *A mother holds her children's hands for a while ... their hearts forever*
> *– Author unknown*

you a stronger person, help you to be more respectful of yourself and others, and increase your sense of self.

When it comes to childbirth, your body will experience a whole range of sensations, from pleasure to pain. However, what is more important is understanding how to work with your body and how your thoughts can impact the mechanics of birth. In addition, learning tools and techniques to help your body's muscles do their job effectively will help you manage and accept the sensations you will experience during birth.

So, my first message to you would be to focus on what you can do to help your body rather than aspire to achieve a pain-free birth.

Will it guarantee you have a "natural birth"?

No.

The term "natural birth" is used and misused a great deal. However, many women are focused on having a birth without medical intervention. The majority of women who follow the techniques in this book will give birth instinctively and intuitively and will not need any additional support or intervention. However, there will be times when some women require additional support. No matter what this support entails, the Natal Hypnotherapy tools and techniques will still help you work with your body and with the medical team around you.

Making a decision to have a child is momentous. It is to decide forever to have your heart go walking around outside your body – Elizabeth Stone

So, what will you learn from reading this book?

As the title suggests, this is a practical guide to birth preparation. This book will help you get rid of the things that hinder the instinctive birth process by helping you to overcome fears and become more confident in your body's ability to give birth. It will help you understand the impact that both your thoughts and the external environment can have on the basic functions of giving birth, as well as the impact they can have on your baby. It will enable you to let go of unhelpful thoughts so that you can let your body give birth instinctively. It will help you tune into your body's natural instincts and abilities.

It is full of practical tips and ideas to help you and your birth partner prepare for a calmer birth, which will most likely lead to your baby having a more relaxed and calmer start in life.

The book is filled with inspiring and heart-warming birth stories and is full of interesting facts on how women have given birth in other cultures. My aim is that, page by page, the things that you are reading will increase your confidence, increase your trust in your body and the process of giving birth, and empower you to feel strong and prepared to have a positive and uplifting birth experience.

A woman's feelings and memories surrounding the birth of her children will stay with her forever. I recently met a woman in her eighties; she could not remember where she had put her glasses, but she could remember every detail and emotion that she had felt when giving birth to her son fifty-five years before.

So much of birth preparation today revolves around the physical and material preparation, and yet very little time and thought are given to emotional or mental preparation for birth. My eighty-year-old friend did not talk about which buggy she had or what colour the nursery was – what she remembered was the birth and how it made her feel.

By reading this book, you are taking a positive step towards truly preparing both your mind and your body for one of the most incredible, powerful and life-changing events. You are giving yourself more choices, teaching yourself more tools and techniques, and helping to Re-frame some of your beliefs about giving birth. Ultimately, you are increasing your trust and confidence that you can influence how you experience birth so that you have an experience which is memorable for all the right reasons.

If you do not get courage from yourself, where then will you go for it?
– Kattrin Davida

Your pregnancy & birth profile

How do you feel about this pregnancy and forthcoming birth?

Throughout your pregnancy, the majority of your antenatal care will be focused on the physical well-being of you and your baby. However, your emotional well-being plays a huge part in your approach to pregnancy and birth. By understanding a bit more about your own feelings, beliefs, hopes and fears, you can begin to separate out those feelings which are useful and beneficial from those which are not useful and do not serve a positive purpose.

So, before you go on any further, get yourself a pen and a cup of something nice and spend some time thinking about each of these questions. You can write them in the book or on a separate piece of paper. However, I would urge you to write them down, as this will encourage age you to be focused, specific and conscious about your feelings and thoughts. It will also help you later on when we go through some of the "letting go" exercises.

Examining how you feel about pregnancy and birth is the first step to accepting and then letting go of any unnecessary or unhelpful thoughts.

Was this a planned pregnancy?

_____

_____

How did you feel about your journey to conception?

_____

_____

_____

_____

_____

A baby is something you carry inside you for nine months, in your arms for three years and in your heart till the day you die – Mary Mason

What were your initial thoughts about being pregnant?

_____

_____

_____

How do you feel now about being pregnant?

_____

_____

_____

_____

_____

_____

What are the three main emotions that you feel when you think about being pregnant and having this baby?

_____

_____

_____

_____

_____

_____

_____

_____

Being a full-time mother is one of the highest-salaried jobs in my field, since the payment is pure love – Mildred B. Vermont

Write down any fears/concerns you have about giving birth. (This is very important, as we will come back to this in more detail later.)

_____

_____

_____

_____

_____

_____

_____

_____

_____

_____

_____

_____

_____

_____

_____

_____

_____

_____

_____

_____

Children and mothers never truly part – bound in the beating of each other's heart
– Charlotte Gray

How do you feel about becoming a mother?

_____

_____

_____

_____

_____

_____

Where are you planning to give birth, and what are the three main reasons for choosing that place?

_____

_____

_____

_____

_____

_____

_____

_____

_____

_____

_____

_____

_____

_____

I never knew how much love my heart could hold until someone called me "mommy"
– Author unknown

Who will be with you during the birth? Why have you chosen them to support you? How well do you think they will be able to support you?

_____

_____

_____

_____

_____

_____

_____

_____

_____

_____

If you know or can find out, what was your own birth like?

_____

_____

_____

_____

_____

_____

_____

_____

_____

_____

_____

_____

If at first you don't succeed, do it the way your mother told you to
— Author unknown

If you have given birth before, write down any negative memories and anything that you would like to change for this forthcoming birth.

_____

_____

_____

_____

_____

_____

_____

_____

_____

_____

_____

_____

Have you ever been to someone else's birth? And, if so, what were your feelings about it?

_____

_____

_____

_____

_____

_____

_____

_____

_____

A mother's arms are made of tenderness and children sleep soundly in them
– Victor Hugo

Write down how you would like the birth of this baby to be.

_____

_____

_____

_____

_____

_____

_____

_____

_____

_____

_____

_____

_____

_____

_____

_____

_____

_____

_____

_____

_____

_____

_____

_____

_____

Mother's love is peace. It need not be acquired, it need not be deserved
– Erich Fromm

_____

_____

_____

_____

_____

_____

_____

_____

_____

_____

_____

_____

_____

_____

_____

_____

_____

_____

_____

_____

_____

_____

_____

_____

_____

_____

_____

_____

_____

_____

_____

The mother's heart is the child's school-room – Henry Ward Beecher

Part 1

Chapter 1 – Mammalising birth

Reproduction is the pinnacle of nature. That is essentially why we are here – to reproduce. In the natural world, male and female are drawn together to reproduce and to continue their species. For men and women the process of reproduction is often one which is sensual, passionate, pleasurable and intimate. It is one in which our bodies know what to do, with no conscious input from ourselves. In the majority of cases, our bodies know how to release eggs and sperm, the sperm know how to find and fertilise an egg, the fertilised egg knows how to divide, and the embryo knows how to draw all it needs from the mother's body and to grow and develop into a perfect human baby.

Did you know?

The word "mammal" comes from the Latin "mamma" meaning breast, derived from the milk production that takes place in female mammals.

This "knowing" comes from our genetic make-up or DNA. For example, the DNA within a woman tells her body how and when to release an egg, to prepare a safe place for the egg to be fertilised and to grow a perfect child. Then the DNA within the baby-to-be provides all the instructions as to when and how to create a heart, toenails, eyelashes, vertebrae, a digestive system, and so on. The DNA in the mother has ensured that the physical structure of her uterus and pelvis is exquisitely designed to change and adapt to accommodate her growing baby. Her brain and body work in complete harmony, producing all the right hormones throughout her pregnancy and leading up to the birth. Once her baby is born, her genetic make-up ensures that her breasts can then provide all the nourishment and immunity that her child needs for the first months and even years of its life.

Did you know?

The Chagga of Tanzania have a saying:

"Pay attention to the pregnant woman – there is no one more important than she."

All the cells and organs within your body were designed to fulfil a function. All the cells in your body have a purpose and instinctively know what to do. No one ever taught you

God could not be everywhere, so he created mothers – Jewish proverb

or your body how to digest food or how to fight off harmful bacteria. Your heart is continually contracting and releasing 24 hours a day. Your digestive system contracts and releases to help food pass through your body. Your large intestine contracts and releases to pass waste products out of your body. The sphincter muscles in your body are held tightly closed until they are ready to release their contents.

All of these functions happen painlessly in a healthy body. Yes, if there is damage or a block of energy from things such as stress, fear or bad eating habits, then even these functions can become painful.

In the same way, your body was designed to birth your baby without severe pain. It is only when there is a block from things such as fear, tension or anxiety that the natural process becomes excessively painful.

So, with such an amazing DNA set-up and such a perfect system, why is it that so many women have lost the belief in their body's ability to give birth?

Why have women lost the trust that they can do it?

What has gone wrong?

What is it about our society that is so different to others, where birth is not viewed with such fear?

We are after all just mammals

Before I go on to answer these questions, it is really useful to take a step back and talk about the basics. Let's stop for a moment to think about who and what we are.

Essentially, you and I are mammals: very sophisticated, well-clothed and clever ones, but just mammals none the less. Our bodies have not really changed in hundreds of thousands of years. The way in which our babies are made and born is the same as it has been since women first walked the earth. Our primal needs and the primal needs of babies are still essentially the same.

Did you know?

All mammals can hold back or bring on labour depending on how safe they feel.

A mother's love for her child is like nothing else in the world. It knows no law, no pity, it dares all things and crushes down remorselessly all that stands in its path –
Agatha Christie

Mammals are characterised by the fact that a female grows her baby within her body; her brain then secretes a number of hormones which trigger and maintain the muscular movements needed to give birth; and she then provides milk for her offspring once they have been born.

This is the same for all mammals.

Have you ever witnessed a mammal give birth in a natural setting?

Maybe you have seen wild animals give birth on a nature programme, or you have taken a sneaky peek at your cat giving birth. Given the right conditions, i.e. an undisturbed natural setting and environment, what are the key characteristics of a mammal's birth experience?

A mum's experience

"I attended a Hypnobirthing course because I was very worried about the birth.

The most important things that I learned were that, like all other mammals, my body knew exactly what to do and that I was able to work with my body and so manage my birth experience. I practised the techniques regularly by listening to the hypnotherapy tracks and always used aromatherapy at the same time (to add another relaxation anchor).

When I went into labour at around 4 a.m., I was able to stay really relaxed and breathe calmly all the time. I stayed at home as long as possible and finally went into hospital at 12.15 a.m. I was sure the midwife was going to send me home, as at first she did not think I was in labour. However, the midwife had a quick check and said: 'You are not going anywhere. You are fully dilated – baby is on his way!!!' Baby Thomas was born at 2.05 p.m.

I cannot thank you enough for the two days I spent on the course with a very nice bunch of couples and an awesome teacher! If I have another baby one day, I will definitely be using Natal Hypnotherapy again! Thank you all."

Sonia Horta, UK

All mothers are working mothers – Author unknown

Mammals that are left to give birth in a natural setting will characteristically:

- Find somewhere safe and quiet
- Usually give birth in the dark
- Appear very relaxed and calm
- Moan quietly and rhythmically

Even though we know that animals feel pain in other situations, during the birth they usually remain quiet and calm and do not appear to show signs that they are in pain (this is not always the case with animals in captivity such as horses or cows, which can show signs of pain and fear).

Mammals will give birth instinctively and without any help. There are some species that will be protected by other members of their group, such as dolphins and elephants, but essentially a birthing mammal will just get on with it, quite often unattended.

As far as we can tell, a mammal does not question what will happen to her during birth. She does not know about the physiological process. She has not watched One Born Every Minute, Discovery Health or Holby City! She simply accepts what happens to her, does not fight it, and lets her body get on with it.

For her it is the same as any other bodily function. When you need to go to the toilet, you do not stop and think about it; you do not ask yourself questions. You simply go somewhere quiet, private and safe. You get into a good position and let your body get on with it: you allow gravity to assist; you work with the natural urge to push; you allow your sphincter muscles to work effectively. Now I am not saying that having a baby is the same as going to the toilet – but it uses the same type of muscles and the same natural ejection reflex which, I am sure you would agree, would be pretty hard to do lying down with a group of people watching you!

There is of course much more involved with giving birth, but, fundamentally, the instinctive response in a mammal is the same for both.

Can mammals influence their own birth?

In essence, a mammal will not give birth if she feels that she is in danger, threatened, observed or disturbed. Somehow a powerful response in her body kicks in to enable her to stop or substantially slow down the labour until she can get somewhere safe and allow the birthing to continue. This is an example of what is known as the "fight or flight" mechanism.

Before becoming a mother I had a hundred theories on how to bring up children. Now I have seven children and only one theory: love them, especially when they least deserve to be loved – Kate Samperi

In researching mammals' birth patterns, it is clear that mammals have some element of control over where and when they give birth. For example, migrating wildebeest will all go into labour and give birth within hours of each other, while the rest of the herd stop and protect the birthing females. For new-world monkeys, early labour can stop at sunrise and resume after sunset, when the group is encamped for the night and the expectant mother will not be distracted by the need to forage. In research trials, pregnant chimpanzees who were being observed did not give birth until the researchers gave up waiting and went home![1]

It should be no surprise, therefore, that, in the same way, women also have this instinctual mechanism to "shut down" or slow down labour if they feel frightened, observed or feel that it is not safe to give birth.

A mum's experience

"After a day or so of mild twinges, I called the hospital to let them know I might be coming in later to have my baby. Whilst chatting to the midwife I had a few more twinges, and by the end of the conversation the midwife told me to come in as soon as I could, as she felt I was probably in labour. I phoned my husband, who was at work, and seven minutes later he was falling through the front door, pulling off his tie and kicking his shoes off; he was panicking much more than me. Half an hour and a few contractions later, we were at the hospital. I was 4 cm. I'd packed my Natal Hypnotherapy music CD but didn't get a chance to put it on, as an hour and forty minutes after arriving at hospital I'd given birth.

However, every time I had a contraction, all I kept thinking about was how I was getting closer and closer to meeting my baby. I kept visualising my older daughter on the shore of a beautiful sandy paradise island, holding a baby, and with every contraction I would ride the crest of a wave which was taking me closer and closer to the two of them. It was WONDERFUL!!! I loved every second of the experience. I made very little noise except for when the baby's head was crowning, when I made the sound of a very large wild animal. As soon as she was born, I said, 'I want another one'; I didn't want it to stop, I was enjoying it all so much!! I can't thank you enough. I have recommended the tracks to EVERY pregnant woman I have met!!"

Sarah Tiffin, UK

A mother's joy begins when new life is stirring inside ... when a tiny heartbeat is heard for the very first time, and a playful kick reminds her that she is never alone. – Author unknown

Imagine yourself as a lone woman labouring in a jungle. Suppose you saw, or even thought you saw, a fierce animal lurking in the nearby shadows. What do you think would happen? Would you have a conscious choice on what happens next? You may think you could control the situation, but your body would already have made the decision. Your labour would slow down or even stop until you could escape and feel safe again, or your baby would be born very quickly so you could pick up your baby and run away to safety.

So, what is the difference between humans and other mammals?

As we know, all mammals share the same physical processes and functions for reproduction – the release and fertilisation of eggs, the release of complex hormones, the contraction of the uterus to birth the baby, and the production of milk. The human body and the human baby have similar physical proportions and ratios to those of other mammals. The strength and ability of the uterine muscles in a woman are similar to those of other female mammals.

So, why is it that a human mother is often perceived to have such excruciating and agonising pain when giving birth, when other mammals do not?

In his book *Birth and Breastfeeding*, Michel Odent (the famous French birth expert who is one of the leading pioneers in reclaiming birth as a natural instinctive process) summarises his 25 years of research:

> *I learned that human beings are mammals. All mammals hide themselves, isolate themselves to give birth. They need privacy. It is the same for humans. We should be aware of this need for privacy.*[2]

However, at the time that he wrote this, many of his colleagues in France claimed that this view was insulting and derogatory, remarking that humans are far better than mammals. We are empowered by language, culture, symbolism, and so on. For example, Fernand Lamaze, the founder of the "Lamaze method", which is very popular in the USA, believed that women needed to be taught to give birth in the same way that we teach children to read or to swim.

In some ways, both Odent and Lamaze were right. The main difference between mammals and humans is that we have developed much larger and more complex brains. We still have the primal part of the brain, which functions in the same way as those in other mammals, but we have also developed the newer part of the brain called the neocortex. It is this part which is responsible for the development of intelligence, analysis, language, inhibitions and irrational fears.

A little girl, asked where her home was, replied, 'Where mother is'
– Keith L. Brooks

It is the stimulus to this part of the brain which causes the human mind to "interfere" with the instinctive birthing process and so lose the ability to completely let go and surrender to the birthing brain. At the top of the list of differences are the emotions of fear and anxiety.

As we have already touched on, fear and anxiety can have a real physical impact on the progress of labour in all mammals.

---

[1] Newton, N., 1971, Interrelationships between various aspects of the female reproductive role, psychosomatic medicine in obstetrics and gynaecology, third congress pp. 338–90.

[2] Odent, M., 2007, *Birth and Breastfeeding*, Clairview Books; 2nd Revised edition.

Mother – that was the bank where we deposited all our hurts and worries
– T. De Witt Talmage

A mum's experience

"What an amazing birth I had! Learning Natal Hypnotherapy gave me strength to trust my body, strength to challenge and stand up for myself when needed, peace when I was not sure, calmness when all I knew was to breathe, and wisdom in knowing women and female mammals before me have all given birth.

On 27 February my hubby wanted to go to trivia evening at 7 p.m., which was fine, as I'd been experiencing little period pains on and off for a while. I would just breathe through them, put on my Natal Hypnotherapy birthing tracks, and lie on the couch, as it was the most comfortable. By 9 p.m. the period pains were a little stronger, lasting 30 to 40 seconds, yet I thought, oh, that's not too bad, I'll just let hubby know to come on home, as I thought maybe I was in labour.

Hubby raced home excited, only to find me lying on the couch, breathing, waiting for the wave to ease up, and then I was up giving him a hug. The contractions stayed constant every 15 mins, 40 to 45 sec. It was like very strong period pains where even your hearing turns off as you centre yourself. I started showering at home, as my lower back started getting achy. It was a hot night and yet the hot water on my lower back was sensational. My mind knew I was in labour, yet at the same time I could talk, walk and then go silent and concentrate when a contraction started. At about 10.45 p.m. we made the first call to the midwife, as I needed to know exactly what was going on, not having waters broken or any 'bloody show'.

The midwife was asleep when we called, drowsy and not very with it. I said 'I think I'm in labour' and told her the times of contractions. We basically had a nice conversation with moments of 'time out' when the contractions took a hold. Yet she didn't think I was in labour, as it was not 'normal' to have those times, no waters breaking, etc. 'Stay put,' she said. 'You're not in labour. Just sit tight and call me back in a couple of hours.'

This was when some of the fear kicked in, which made contractions stronger! Someone doubting me because what I was going through was not normal. I went back to the couch and focused on my Natal Hypnotherapy breathing and just listening to my breath. I really didn't have a special place to go – my nostrils were my special place where my breath felt warm, safe and certain.

I started talking about maybe needing drugs; if the midwife didn't think I was in labour, then I didn't want to be in much more discomfort [self-doubt phase]. My husband, being the charmer, went, 'What? After all your talk of strength and woman wisdom you want drugs? Go and listen to the English woman on those tracks!". I did and whimpered at how I could have felt so weak as to want drugs just then.

Back in the shower I decided to have a feel, as I was feeling quite a lot of pressure down below. I could feel what I thought was a head. I got hubby to check – yep, it was a head. We then got excited and at 11.55 p.m. called the midwife, who still insisted I was not in labour, but said that if we wanted to go to the hospital the staff would check me out and then send me home ... 'Get me to the hospital darling!!!'

Taxi we did! One of the most uncomfortable rides of my life, although the driver of the cab was excellent – 'Don't worry, madam, my wife has had three children.' Two contractions and we were at the front of the hospital. Got out of the cab and vomited – thank goodness I remembered to take an ice-cream bucket. Four old smoking patients congratulated me as I waddled in. A nurse greeted us on the fifth floor, where I once again vomited. Take an ice-cream bucket just in case, gals!

Lying on the bed on my side I had three more contractions. The nurse took forever. She asked me to lie on my back – arrgghh. How on earth have generations of women managed to give birth on their backs????? I had a contraction as she was checking me out and it was THE most awful of all the contractions I experienced. The nurse said, 'Oh, lovey, you're 8.5 cm dilated. Your baby is on its way.' Thank God someone now believed me.

Yey, our buboo was on the way! It was at this point that I wished my mother was alive to give me a hug that only mothers know best. My husband was excellent from 12.30 a.m. to 3.31 a.m.! Showering on a ball, birthing pool (which I didn't like that much), finally on all fours leaning into a beanbag.

As I was resting, the midwife leaned in and said, 'Maria, I have to give you antibiotics because last time you were in I forgot to tell you that you have the strep B...' Or whatever it's called ... Well, this wakes me up from my resting period. The lioness in me grrrrssss! 'Nope, not having it,' I said. She explained to me that my waters had still not broken and that the baby might be at risk.

My intuition was strong and in tune, and knew that the baby was safe. I reluctantly agreed to have the drip in, which meant no labouring for 2hrs ... Half an hour later, mother nature decided that it was just too bad – the baby was coming out. The *midwife agreed, telling me to push. Well, I tell you what – it's like pushing the biggest poo you've ever done out.*

The best thing my husband did was place a very warm cloth over the perineum, which was heavenly soothing. Make sure your hubbies do this for you, as I believe it relaxed me more and left me with no tearing! Once I got that head out I took a small break. The midwife commanded me to push again; somehow the strength to push came from nowhere. Then, pop – out came the shoulder, and then the rest of the body. The little baby was still in its sack!!! The baby stretched and broke itself out and there before my eyes was our beautiful new baby girl. I think I then went into bliss shock!

There was very little bleeding, no tearing, no drugs. The pushing out of the placenta was very easy and was out in one last strong push, no discomfort! We had the birth centre to ourselves for two nights and were then home again. We played the Natal Hypnotherapy birthing music to ease all of us into our new life.

What an amazing journey I'd just been on!! I'm not scared at all anymore and am empowered. We had very little support around us. No mother, a mother-in-law who did not agree, and many, many friends who found us suddenly 'strange'. I had to believe in myself and believe in hundreds of years of women birthing by themselves.

Thank you for creating such wonderfully empowering tracks for women.

They gave me strength to trust my body, strength to challenge and stand up for myself when needed, peace when I was not sure, calmness when all I knew was to breathe, and wisdom in knowing women and female mammals before me have all given birth. I loved birthing and would love to be able to learn Natal Hypnotherapy to help empower mothers-to-be to trust in themselves. Congratulations to you all! With thanks."

Maria Walker, Brisbane, Australia

Chapter 2 – Instinctive birthing

Before we explore the impact that fear has on giving birth, it is useful to understand what happens, from a physical, hormonal and emotional perspective, when a woman gives birth instinctively.

It is the most dramatic event that can take place in the human body and involves an amazing cocktail of hormones, muscular changes, movements of body parts, changes in the shape and size of muscles, emotional, mental and physical changes, intense sensations and uncontrollable urges. As renowned midwife and author Ina May Gaskin says:

It is the Mount Everest of physical functions in a mammal.[1]

If you had never seen it before you would not think it possible, and yet it happens thousands of times every day and has done for millions of years.

As you are already aware, nature designed birth to be a calm and manageable experience for an animal left alone. Having said that, the following is also true for most women:

Yes, giving birth is hard work.
Yes, giving birth is intense.
Yes, you will feel strong sensations in your uterus.
Yes, there will be times when you wonder if you can cope.

However, your state of mind and physical well-being will play an important role in how well you respond to the process. It is a bit like running a marathon: if you go into it unprepared, dreading it and feeling certain that you will not make it all the way, the chances are that you won't.

However, if you are mentally and physically fit, practise, warm up your muscles, pace yourself and visualise yourself crossing the finishing line, you probably will. It will still be hard work – you will use a lot of energy, your muscles will feel the strain and you may finish exhausted – but you will still be able to enjoy it and feel great at the end.

It was when I had my first child that I understood how much my mother loved me –
from "For Mother – A Bouquet of Sentiments"

When it comes to giving birth, one of the most fundamental factors in having an instinctive birth is that you reduce stimulation of your neocortex or higher intelligence (more on that later) and hand control over to your birthing brain. By going into the birth feeling positive, prepared and confident, you are far more likely to manage the sensations and stay in control of how you respond to the environment around you, thus flowing through the birthing process.

When left alone, nature works wonderfully well, as the birthing process is usually long enough and gradual enough to allow the mother to adapt to the changes within her body. As the birthing process and the sensations become more intense, they increase the mother's focus and ability to "close down" all other parts of herself, so channelling all her energy to her birthing body.

Key signs that labour is imminent

In the last few weeks and days of pregnancy, there are several signs which indicate that your baby is getting ready to be born:

- Most babies are born head first. In the last few weeks of pregnancy, the baby will drop further down into your pelvis (called "being engaged"). You will feel more pressure in the lowest part of your stomach and pelvis and may feel you have a little more room to breathe.

- You may experience an increase in vaginal mucus and will feel quite "wet".

- Your body may release the mucus plug from your cervix (sometimes called a "show"), which has protected the uterus from infection during pregnancy. It will be pinkish in colour and may have a little blood. This release can continue over a few days and indeed throughout the birth.

- You may have a runny bowel movement. The digestive system uses up a great deal of energy and so, as labour is about to start, the body does not want to worry about digesting food. As a result you naturally expel any waste product from the body, which also helps to make more room for the baby to be born.

A baby has a special way of adding joy in every single day – Author unknown

- Your blood pressure may go up a bit – this is a sign that your body is getting on with things behind the scenes.

- "Waters breaking" – this is a strange term used to denote the rupture of the membrane holding the baby and amniotic fluid in. This can release a little or a lot of the fluid. However, it is important to remember that your body will continue to produce amniotic fluid, so there is no worry that the baby will go "dry".

- Practice contractions – for weeks leading up to the birth of the baby, your uterus will be having lots of practice or warm-up contractions (Braxton Hicks). These are helping the muscle fibres of the uterus to tone and the cervix to soften and get ready to open. Many women confuse Braxton Hicks for real contractions and often wonder if they are actually in labour or not.

How will you know you are in labour?

This is a difficult one, as, put quite simply, "when you are you will know". Usually the pattern and frequency of Braxton Hicks changes to become steadier and follow a regular and more rhythmical pattern. The uterus becomes hard during a contraction, especially at the top – you can visibly see when you are having one through your stomach and back muscles. If you are in active labour, then lying down or going for a walk will not stop the contractions, which often happens with Braxton Hicks. Your mood and emotional state will change, too. (More of this will be explained later.)

No one knows exactly what triggers birth; however, it is strongly believed that, when the baby is ready, a message is sent through to the brain to begin the production of the cocktail of hormones for birth.

Birthing begins when the hormone oxytocin is released. This hormone triggers the muscles of the uterus to begin to flex and tighten, known as a contraction. The uterus is the largest bag of muscles in your body and is made up of circular muscles at the bottom, known as the cervix, and longitudinal muscles running down from the top.

Did you know?

Your metabolism rate increases by 25% late in your pregnancy, so your body is 25% more efficient in converting nutrients into energy.

No one knows how children will turn out; a great tree often springs from a tender plant – Norwegian proverb

The longitudinal muscles are soft and supple and reach down to draw back the circular muscles at the bottom gently, just like slowly pulling a polo-neck jumper over your head. When the muscles flex, you feel them as a warm sensation or "the burn", just like you do with intense exercise, such as when you stay in a half-squat position for some time and can really feel the muscles heat up in your thighs.

If all the other muscles around the uterus are soft and relaxed, then there is no resistance or strain and the opening of the round muscles can be done freely and comfortably.

The physical journey of birth

These movements of the muscles in the uterus slowly and gradually build up in frequency and length as the birth progresses. Unlike running a marathon, nature was kind enough to always give you a rest between contractions; so, contrary to the myth that you are in labour for hours on end, your muscles are only contracting for about a minute at a time, followed by several minutes' rest.

Once the round muscles or the cervix are fully open, the hormone relaxin helps the muscles in the birth canal fan open. These muscles are usually ridged or are like a concertina, so, given the right conditions, these muscles can spread out and expand to be large enough for a baby to pass through. As the round muscles of the cervix are pulled up into the long muscles of the uterus, the baby's passage way becomes clear.

Once this happens, the body steps up a gear and the long muscles begin to push the baby down into the birth canal. This urge to bear down, or "foetal ejection reflex", is a natural, instinctive reflex – similar to coughing or sneezing. It is almost impossible to ignore, and to many women it can feel almost pleasurable after the tightening and releasing sensations.

It is really important to know that there can often be a lull or gap in, or simply a slowing down of, the contractions between

Did you know?

Most cultures believe that the placenta has a spiritual or physical significance and the majority bury the placenta. The Maori word for placenta is Whenna which also means "earth". The Tolong of the Philippines place the placenta in a clay pot, smoke it and then bury it.

The Bukinon of the Philippines consider the placenta "the brother" of the baby. They bury the placenta under the house and believe that the spirit of the placenta returns to the sky.

A baby is sunshine and moonbeams – brightening your world as never before
– Author unknown

the passage way being clear (known as fully dilated) and experiencing the ejection reflex – this is sometimes referred to as the "rest and be thankful" phase.

During this time, your baby is getting into the right position and your body is taking a well-earned rest before the final part of the birth. By trusting your body and allowing the urge to bear down to come naturally, your body will do the rest. It is important not to be hurried into pushing, as research has shown that forced pushing has no benefits to mum or baby[2]. Once the urge is there, your focus should be on listening to your body, breathing deeply and going with the sensations – your body will do the rest.

A mum's experience

"I learnt Natal Hypnotherapy for my second pregnancy – for the birth of my son, I had been induced and, although it wasn't the horrendous experience some people have, I was keen to have a more natural and instinctive labour second time around. The overriding feeling I remember from my first birth was that of being afraid – afraid of the pain, afraid of giving birth, and a general feeling of being out of control.

The second time around, I wanted to be able to trust my instincts, to feel more confident in my body's ability to give birth, to feel in control and to manage the Pain.

Once labour started, my husband took me straight to hospital. I'd asked for the pool to be filled up, as I wanted to have a water birth, but there wasn't enough time! The contractions were very strong, but I somehow felt able to cope with the pain, and even refused gas and air, as I felt it would distract me from giving birth.

Within thirty minutes of arriving at the hospital I was ready to push – I felt the pushing to be very instinctive and so much easier than last time. Unlike my first labour, where I pushed for over an hour, my baby was born less than fifteen minutes later. I had no pain relief and no stitches, and I am convinced that this was mainly due to the beneficial effect of the Natal Hypnotherapy."

Christine Lane, UK

Babies are a link between angels and man – Author unknown

Once the baby has moved down through the birth canal, the usually thick layer of concertina-like muscles of the perineum gradually flatten out and cover a much wider area just as the baby is coming out. In addition, the pressure of the baby's head on the perineum reduces circulation, which helps to numb the area, just like when you sit on your leg for too long and it goes all numb. Again, nature is incredible, as the cells of the perineum have more elasticity than any other part of the body and are flooded with the hormone relaxin to enable them to fan open in order to allow the baby to pass through.

Remarkably, the baby's head is actually designed to reduce in size as the plates in the skull overlap and the baby's head becomes more oval-shaped – so, again, contrary to popular belief, the head is not round but is more the shape of the opening of the vagina. As the baby is descending, the pelvic bones also soften and widen (even more so if you are in a squatting position or upright).

Once the baby has been born, the uterus changes once again and immediately begins to contract down, starting the journey of going back to being a small, hollow, pear-shaped organ. As the uterus shrinks down, the small blood vessels which connect the placenta to the mother get cut off and so the placenta shears away from the edge of the uterus. Once the placenta is no longer attached, the uterus gently expels the placenta, often with one or two pushes from the mother.

So, put in its simplest terms, given the right cocktail of hormones and the right mental, physical and emotional state of the mother, the long muscles of the uterus pull open the round muscles until the passage way is large enough for the baby to slip down and out of the woman's body.

What is also amazing to know is that the muscles of the uterus will work for you no matter what you do. Even if a woman were unconscious or in a coma, the muscles of the uterus would birth her baby.

Babies are bits of stardust, blown from the hand of God – Barretto

Sphincter law

You may be wondering what this title is all about! Well, this is something I learned about from an amazing midwife from the US called Ina May Gaskin. She has been supporting women through birth for decades and has made a fabulous observation about the way our bodies respond to certain environmental situations.

So this is her "sphincter law":

The body has several sphincter muscles – the bladder, rectum, uterus and cervix – which are basically circular muscles whose sole purpose is to hold something in until there is a trigger to open and let things out. Usually this happens when there is sufficient pressure on the circular muscles for them to move apart and so empty or expel the contents. When this happens, the round muscles relax and expand (as much as is needed) to allow the contents to fall out.

Now what is interesting is that these sphincter muscles all have several characteristics in common:

- Sphincters work best in an atmosphere of intimacy, calm and privacy – e.g., would you be able to do a poo in a public toilet without a lock?

- Sphincters cannot be opened at will and do not respond to commands, e.g. "push" or "relax"

- Sphincters involuntarily close if the person feels scared, embarrassed, interrupted or self-conscious

- Relaxation of the mouth and jaw directly correlate to the relaxation of the sphincter muscles in the vagina and anus – laughing is a great way of relaxing these muscles. Ever laughed so much you have wet yourself?

- When the person is stressed the sphincter muscles can also tense up

A classic example of the influence that a person's thoughts and psychology can have over a sphincter muscle was a research study into the areas of the brain which were activated when a person's bladder was opened. The research failed, as it required the participants to urinate whilst being watched and monitored – the participants found it really difficult and unnatural to urinate whilst being observed and so the research was abandoned.

It is the nature of babies to be in bliss – Deepak Chopra

Sphincters have a mind of their own. They can suddenly slam shut if the person becomes frightened or disturbed – men in public toilets will be able to relate to this!

In the same way, an animal will stop birthing and move to a safe place if there is a predator or if they do not feel safe. Humans are the same; we just do not always understand the evolutionary wisdom behind it.

One of the areas of difficulty with the modern approach to birthing is that in many hospitals women are coached in when and how to push. Unfortunately, a sphincter muscle does not respond well to that kind of instruction and can simply tense up or clam shut. Given time and patience, the body will bring about the ejection reflex and there will be the overwhelming urge to bear down as your baby moves through the birth canal.

Ina May tells a story of a woman who was transferred from a home birth to hospital, following medical complications, when she was 7 cm dilated. She was met by a rude, abrupt

A mum's experience

"After a difficult first birth, I was determined that things were going to be different second time around. I was so relaxed in my home environment, with gentle music playing, essential oils burning and candles. I hardly experienced any pain at all, so when the midwife examined me, I was sure that she'd say I had a long way to go. I was really shocked and delighted when she told me I was already 8–9 cm dilated! The whole process lasted only three-and-a-half hours and the midwives just kept commenting on how 'chilled out' I was.

I was laughing and joking right up until about the last thirty minutes, and my toddler slept soundly above us all the way through. At the end, I did ask for gas and air, but I found that it just got in the way of my breathing, so I actually used very little of it. When it was time to push, I gave it everything I'd got. It was all over in less than ten minutes. I had listened to the track at least once a day from about thirty weeks and I'm convinced that it was the main reason why I was so at ease. Using the track made my home birth an amazing, pleasurable experience – so much so that I actually want to do it again! Thank you."

Kate Harris, UK

A father's goodness is higher than the mountain, a mother's goodness deeper than the sea – Japanese proverb

obstetrician, who examined her roughly and painfully, saying that in fact she was only 4 cm. Even though the woman's intellectual mind knew that she was in hospital for a good reason and that the obstetrician was there to help her, her cervix's "mind" simply saw him as an intruder and a predator. As a result her cervix had quickly retracted, as her birthing body had felt that it was not safe to be open and birth her baby. Ina May examined her again and sure enough she was only 4 cm – her cervix had contracted back down.

This is a little-known and often-unrecognised fact amongst obstetricians, doctors and even many midwives: that it is entirely possible for a cervix to close as well as open during labour.

The importance of hormones during labour

When a woman is giving birth, all the activities within her body are dictated by the secretion of hormones. As Ina May Gaskin points out, there is an intricate and exquisitely balanced combination of hormones necessary to trigger all functions of labour and birth[3].

During this time the body releases a complex cocktail of hormones which are vital in order for the "normal" process of birth to be allowed to flow unhindered. These hormones are made in the deepest, most primitive part of our brain and are the same as those secreted by other mammals. Understanding the roles of these hormones and their importance will help you to work with your body more effectively.

When all the birthing hormones are present, the body will go through every detailed stage of labour with no interference or need for anything outside her body, i.e. medical support or intervention.

It is therefore sad and quite worrying that, in modern society, women all over the world are regularly giving birth without the natural secretion of birthing hormones. Instead they are being pumped full of chemical, synthesised hormones to "force" the body to go through the birthing process. These artificial hormones (often made from animal products including horse and pig semen!) create similar physical functions in the body, causing the longitudinal muscles of the uterus to contract and pull up. However, they cannot cross into the brain and so do not trigger the pituitary gland to secrete the additional cocktail of beneficial hormones which enable the body and mind to work with the contractions.

What good mothers and fathers instinctively feel like doing for their babies is usually best after all – Benjamin Spock

Michel Odent asks the question – what will happen to the genetic make-up of the female birthing woman if many generations go by without her using, stimulating and producing the vitally important cocktail of hormones?[4]

Not only do the hormones create the physical functions of birth – that is, the movement of muscles, the relaxing of ligaments, the expanding of the birth canal, and so on – they also have an enormous impact on the emotional and mental state of the mother, especially where bonding and love are concerned.

Oxytocin

This is the queen of all hormones – if you could bottle oxytocin, you would probably become extremely rich. The word oxytocin is derived from the Greek words *okus* and *tokos* meaning quick childbirth[5]. The hormone is nature's way of ensuring the survival of the species, as it is a wonderful incentive to continue to procreate. Oxytocin produces in us such powerful and positive feelings that it has been named as the "hormone of love" by Michel Odent:

> *Whatever facet of love we consider, oxytocin is involved[6].*

It is the hormone which is released whenever the chemical response of "love" kicks in: during love-making, birth, breastfeeding, bonding, cuddling and so on. It truly is the X factor that drives males and females together and that keeps them together. And as it is not a "one-hit wonder", the more oxytocin we have in our system, the more we produce and the better we feel. In research it has been shown to have a cumulative effect, so, the more frequently we are exposed to oxytocin, the longer the effect lasts.

Did you know?

In many cultures, nipple stimulation is used as a means to speed up labour as it releases oxytocin into the system and so encourages contractions.

The production of oxytocin leads to feelings of calm, well being, patience, increased social behaviour, lower blood pressure, better digestion and better healing. It even makes breastfeeding mothers more tolerant of monotony, and thus better able to cope with the challenges of early motherhood.

Oxytocin is present at every point in the reproductive cycle and throughout our lives. It is a rush of oxytocin that stimulates the sexual organs, that causes ejaculation and that causes the cervix to vacuum-in sperm. It causes uterine contractions during orgasm,

Our most basic instinct is not for survival but for family – Paul Pearshall

which not only help the sperm on their way, but also produce a wonderful feeling and sense of well-being[7].

During pregnancy, oxytocin levels are low, but they begin to increase towards the end of the last trimester. High levels of oestrogen at the end of pregnancy increase the number of oxytocin receptors in the mother's brain in readiness to promote maternal behaviour. This means that by the time your baby is born, your brain has been "hard wired" for maternal instincts. During pregnancy, oxytocin triggers frequent uterine contractions, which help to strengthen the uterus and maintain the pregnancy, stimulating the flow of blood from the placenta to the baby. These are often known as "Braxton Hicks" contractions.

Even though no one is exactly sure how labour is triggered, we do know that it is oxytocin which is the "driver" behind labour. It is the pulsating release of oxytocin which triggers the long muscles of the uterus to reach down and gently pull open the circular muscles of the cervix. As the uterus contracts, signals are sent to the brain to produce more oxytocin, which helps the uterus contract more effectively, thus making more oxytocin, and so on. This wonderful cycle of triggers and hormone production will continue throughout labour, as long as the mother is not disturbed.

A mum's experience

"I had a wonderful home birth for my first son. My waters broke at 7 a.m. and my contractions started straight away. The midwife turned up at about 10 a.m., when my contractions were very painful and about five minutes apart. I breathed through all the sensations as the track suggested. I felt in control 97% of the time. I had a few contractions whilst standing, which were much harder to deal with, but I didn't make a sound, except for heavy breathing, until my son was born at 4.32 p.m.

I have recommended Natal Hypnotherapy to many of my friends and believe I would have been a total wreck had I not had them for support. The concept that being scared increases adrenalin, which affects oxytocin etc, made it very easy for me to understand that I had to be calm throughout. Thank you."

Emma Lyman, UK

Family life is a bit like a runny peach pie – not perfect, but who's complaining?
– Robert Brault

During labour, oxytocin receptors throughout the body are on high alert. These receptors are found in the cervix, birth canal, perineum, vagina and nipples, and even in the skin. Gentle pressure, massage and stimulation in any of these areas (the release of oxytocin during massage is well reported[8]) ensure that the production of oxytocin will remain steady and high, as long as there is no interference from fear-induced adrenalin, drugs or artificial hormones.

Once the gap in the cervix is large enough for the baby to pass through, and the head begins to press down into the birth canal, the receptors there send a new wave of signals, which trigger another surge of oxytocin, as the force of the contractions changes to one of pushing down rather than opening the cervix.

As well as the physical effects, oxytocin helps a woman to mentally "go off to a different plane" or "go into the zone" so that she lets go on a psychological, as well as a physiological, level, allowing her body to take control[9].

At the moment of birth, if it is undisturbed, unobserved and there is minimal interference, a woman will experience a higher level of oxytocin in her body than at any other time. The reasons for this are manifold. Firstly, it is designed to produce an overwhelming feeling of love towards the baby, facilitating the process of "falling in love". Again, nature is very clever, as this wonderful feeling is a powerful incentive and driver for a mother to look after her baby.

On a physical level, this oxytocin sends signals to the brain to begin producing milk for the baby, whilst also triggering the uterus to begin to shrink back down again to its pre-pregnancy shape and size and to release the placenta. Skin-to-skin contact with your baby and the massaging movements of your baby's hands as she finds her way to the breast add to the stimulation to produce even more oxytocin. It is not a coincidence that there is a high concentration of oxytocin receptors in the skin of your chest, meaning that placing your baby on your chest will trigger even more oxytocin – ever wondered why hugging feels so good?

During this time it is vital that the mother and baby are left undisturbed, with as little stimulation as possible. It is also very important to keep the room really warm, as being cold can inhibit the production of oxytocin.

In the weeks after the birth of the baby, oxytocin continues to play a vital role in the production of prolactin (hormone for producing milk) and of course in the bonding process. As well all the emotional benefits from oxytocin, such as having a sense of calm, well-being and patience, breastfeeding women also benefit from physical changes, including increased functioning of the digestive tract, so that they digest food effectively and efficiently in order to

Parenthood is a lot easier to get into than out of – Bruce Lansky

produce the right amount of milk for their baby, and the increased ability of the body to heal itself.

The production of oxytocin is not a conscious one – that is to say, it is not one that can be controlled by our higher intelligence. Oxytocin is a very instinctive and powerful, yet very sensitive, hormone. Any disturbance or interference – such as fear, embarrassment, feeling observed, feeling cold, or being exposed to loud noises – can slow down or even stop the production of oxytocin. Any overstimulation of the neocortex (the higher-intelligence part of us, which makes us different from mammals), such as talking, questions, analysing, form-filling, etc., can have a similar effect. In addition, medical interventions such as induction, epidurals, anaesthetic injections or episiotomy will seriously scare off this wonderful hormone.

There may be times when the release of oxytocin is disturbed; however, the Natal Hypnotherapy skills that you will learn later in this book will enable you to deal with such interruptions or disturbances, so that you can quickly and easily get back on track to an instinctive birth.

I hope you can see just how important this wonderful hormone is and that, from now on, you will make it a priority to create the right environment and the physical and mental conditions to ensure that you produce bucketfuls during the birth and once the baby has been born.

Oxytocin, though, does not work in isolation. It is the production of an intricate cocktail of hormones which enables the body to open and release your baby.

Other important hormones include:

Endorphins

Endorphins are the body's natural painkillers or opiates. Endorphins are released when the body is involved with physical activity and especially when there is a level of discomfort or pain; for example, when running or exercising hard, the muscles begin to ache and the body produces endorphins.

Scientists discovered endorphins ("endogenous morphine") in the mid-'70s, and found that neurotransmitters in the brain have pain-relieving properties similar to

Did you know?

In Bangladesh, massage by the Daia or midwife is considered to be the best form of pain relief, as it provides constant physical and emotional support.

I think, at a child's birth, if a mother could ask a fairy godmother to endow it with the most useful gift, that gift would be curiosity – Eleanor Roosevelt

morphine. When endorphins attach to opiate receptor neurons, they reduce the intensity of pain in the human body by naturally blocking pain signals produced by the nervous system.

During the birth, the flow of the oxytocin triggers the flow of endorphins, which gradually increase as the labour progresses. By the time the baby is ready to be born, a woman's body is so full of endorphins that many of the sensations are naturally numbed.

This hormone actually blocks the pain impulses reaching the brain, thus making the perception of pain far less intense. Endorphins are also released when a woman is massaged during labour.

Endorphins offer a number of benefits for pregnant and birthing women:

- They are natural painkillers, produced in response to the heavy work of pregnancy and the stress of uterine contractions.

- They create a sense of well-being and promote positive feelings.

- They offer a natural reward for the effort involved in giving birth.

Relaxin

This hormone is secreted during pregnancy, again building up to a maximum during the birth. It is a wonderful hormone, as it helps to make all the ligaments, muscles and tissues soft, supple and stretchy. It helps to soften and relax the ligaments and muscles in the pelvis and the perineum, allowing the bones to shift to accommodate the baby; it helps the uterus to become evenly smooth as it expands to accommodate the baby; and it helps to soften the round muscles of the cervix.

During the birth, the more a mother breathes in plenty of oxygen and stays relaxed, the higher the levels of relaxin, which help the birth canal to soften and widen in order to allow the baby to pass through.

Prostaglandin

This is the hormone that helps the cervix to soften and spread out. The body will produce this hormone in the weeks leading up to the birth.

Semen is a natural carrier of prostaglandin and so making love in the build-up to giving birth can help to soften the cervix.

A ship under sail and a big-bellied woman are the handsomest two things that can be seen – Benjamin Franklin

Environmental factors

As we have just explored, one of the most important factors in ensuring an instinctive birth is to help facilitate the natural production of birthing hormones. Fundamentally, this can be done by letting go of fears, trusting your body and handing control over to your birthing brain. However, the environment in which you give birth will also play an important role in helping to produce the right hormones.

Remember the environmental conditions chosen by mammals when they give birth?

They will usually choose somewhere safe, dark and private. In a similar way, if you look at many traditional cultures, women often choose a specific location for the birth of their babies. They usually choose a place in which they feel safe, private, warm and dark, such as a birthing hut or even inside a hollowed-out tree, such as the Hadza in Tanzania[10].

It is interesting to note that the optimum conditions for giving birth mirror the optimum conditions for conceiving a baby. During love-making, the woman's body produces high levels of oxytocin as long as she feels safe, private, warm and unobserved. The more relaxed and confident she is, the more enjoyable and ultimately successful the experience will be.

So, whether you choose to give birth at home or in hospital, there are certain things that you can do to facilitate the most natural and comfortable birth. Here are a few basic guidelines, which all revolve around enabling a birthing woman to remain "primal".

- **Privacy**
  A birthing mother should not feel observed (and this includes using cameras, videos and foetal monitors), as this can increase her levels of anxiety, inhibitions and an expectation to "perform". As Michel Odent points out: *"we all feel differently when we are being observed ... privacy is a factor which facilitates the reduction of the neocortical control"*[11]

Just think, how easy would it be for you to fall asleep knowing people are watching you?

It is therefore not surprising that many women who go into hospital to give birth choose to spend time in the bathroom or the toilet, where they can close or even lock the door and be left alone.

I will love the light for it shows me the way. Yet I will endure the darkness for it shows me the stars – Og Mandino

- **Safety**

As we will see later, if a woman feels anxious or scared, her body will not be able to birth effectively. Therefore, as far as possible, choose to give birth in a place where you feel safe and well cared for and aim to reduce all potential concerns and anxieties.

- **Quiet**

When a woman is in established labour, it is important that she is able to focus inwards and is not distracted by noises around her. To help her become more "primal", it is important not to stimulate the neocortex. Simply asking her a question can bring her out of her "zone" and so disrupt the hormonal dance of labour. Even though she may appear to be "away with the fairies", she will still be able to hear everything around her and so any unnecessary or disruptive conversation may disturb her.

Tip: You may like to suggest that during a contraction everyone is silent to allow you to focus and work with your body.

- **Low lights**

Bright lights are stimulating and can be intimidating, as they naturally increase the flow of adrenalin. In addition, a woman in a brightly lit room may feel more observed. As with all mammals, a birthing mother will feel calmer, safer and more private if the lights are dimmed.

- **Warmth**

The temperature is also important. If a mother gets cold, she will start to produce adrenalin and will divert blood away from the uterus in order to maintain her body temperature.

If you are going into hospital or to a birth centre, here are a few things you can do to create the best environment for birth:

1. Bring your own duvet or blanket

What does your duvet represent to you? Comfort, safety, warmth, privacy. You can hide under your duvet and disappear into your own world no matter what is going on around you.

Did you know?

The Hadza tribe in Tanzania choose to give birth inside a huge hollowed-out tree called the Baobab tree. They go into the tree alone and do not come out for many days after the birth of their baby.

Child-rearing myth #1: Labour ends when the baby is born – Anonymous

2. Earplugs or earphones
You can use these to block out any noise and so stay focused.

3. Eye mask
If you are giving birth during the day and want to make your space a little darker, bring in an eye mask.

4. Turn off lights and close curtains
You can switch on an angle poise lamp and turn it towards the wall to get a small amount of diffused light. Many midwives are happy to use a torch in a darkened room so that they can see what is happening without disturbing the mother. You can also bring in electric tea lights which give off a small candle-like light but without the flame.

5. 'Do not disturb' sign
Place a sign outside the door asking not to be disturbed and for anyone to knock and then wait to be invited in.

6. Cover up unnecessary equipment
Throw a sheet or blanket over any medical/clinical equipment to help make your space more comforting and homely.

The emotional map of birth

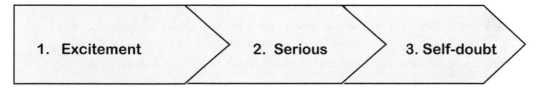

1. Excitement   2. Serious   3. Self-doubt

The journey to birth can be assessed in several ways. The traditional medical approach uses time and dilation as key measurements. However, every woman is unique and her birthing should not routinely be set against a clock. In fact, it is the use of the clock in labour which probably leads to more intervention than any other instrument.

Using internal examinations is another method used to assess the labour, but again the level of dilation has no real bearing on the progress of the birth. Women can be 2–3 cm dilated for days or can go from 3 cm to fully dilated within an hour and can even go from 6 cm to 3 cm (see sphincter law).

Having a baby is like falling in love again, both with your husband and your child –
Tina Brown

A far better way to assess the progress is by being aware of the emotional map of birth coupled with the length of, and the time between, contractions. When you assess all three together you will have a clearer idea of where in the birthing process you are.

We have identified three main emotional phases that almost all women go through during labour:

Phase 1. Excitement phase

Things are beginning! You have noticed changes in the feeling and frequency of the tightenings in your stomach. They are coming more regularly and lasting 30–45 seconds.

What should you do during this phase?

If things feel like they are starting for real and it is during the day, then this is the time for you to carry on your daily business. You can often just ignore the contractions or you can pause

A mum's experience

"After an extremely painful and super-fast labour with my first baby (three-and-a-half hours), I knew I had to overcome the memories of pain which were stressing me out as my second labour drew near, so I began listening to the birth preparation track.

On my due date I started getting period-style cramps – things were starting, but I was so chilled and if anything really excited! Using my breathing and relaxing techniques from the track I went into a more serious meditative state but was still fully
aware of what was going on around me – just really enjoying the peaceful state. Labour progressed calmly and, dare I say it, I actually looked forward to the contractions, as the peace that followed was sublime – the climb down from a contraction was bliss!! So strange – I never thought it possible. My husband, midwife and mother were in shock at how calmly those five hours went!! The pushing stage was hard but I pushed four times and he was out – Zac was born at 3 p.m. HAPPY MAMA, thanks so much."

Amina Jamil, UK

I thought my mom's whole purpose was to be my mom. That's how she made me feel
– Natasha Gregson Wagner

what you are doing briefly by relaxing, and breathing steadily and deeply, allowing the abdomen to remain loose and floppy. This is actually a good time to do something active such as go for a walk, watch a film, go out for dinner, go shopping, and so on.

It is a good idea to think of a specific plan or project in advance of going into labour which you are going to keep just for this time – it may be to bake a birthday cake for your baby; it may be to watch a favourite film; or it may be to cut a special arrangement of flowers from the garden.

During this time, all sorts of things are changing inside your body. Your baby may be getting into a better position, and the long firm "neck" of the uterus or cervix needs to soften, thin out and be pulled back up into your uterus before it can actually start to open.

For a first-time mum, this initial stage can go on for a very long time, so it is important that you do not take it too seriously and get into your birthing mode too soon. If you can sleep, then that is great, or at least go to bed and rest during contractions. If it is "real" labour, it will not stop by lying down.

A very wise old midwife once told me that if things start in the evening, take a couple of paracetamol or a stiff drink and go to sleep. Don't be shocked – remember that many women are happy to have opiates pumped into their bodies during labour, so a good whisky at this stage of your pregnancy will not do any harm.

It is especially important to avoid going into hospital too soon, as you are likely to be sent home, which can feel demoralising or scary, or you will become open to more intervention, as the clock will start ticking as soon as you arrive at hospital. If you do have an internal examination during this time it is so important not to focus on the number of centimetres dilated you are. Many women feel disheartened if they are examined and are pronounced to be 2 or 3 cm after many, many hours of contractions.

Did you know?

In some tribal societies in New Guinea, they have no idea how long pregnancy should last, and believe that the child will be born any time it decides is right.

Remember that every movement in your body serves a purpose, and it is only our intellectual brain that thinks numbers are important. What is more important than numbers is trusting and believing that your body is moving, shifting, softening, tightening and relaxing to get ready for your cervix to open and release your baby.

Now, as always, the most automated appliance in a household is the mother
– Beverly Jones

Phase 2. Serious phase

The serious part is when you are in active labour – usually you will have got to the 3 cm hurdle and your cervix will now be beginning to open or dilate, rather than softening and thinning. At this point you feel like you are really getting on with the business of birthing. Excitement gives way to concentration and seriousness. By this point contractions will be 45–60 seconds long and 3–5 minutes apart.

You will begin to feel the need to rest, lie or sit down between each contraction and then move into a comfortable position for the contraction itself. These are good, powerful and effective contractions. You will now need to concentrate heavily on your breathing and use different coping strategies, including relaxation and visualisation techniques. You will become totally absorbed and not want to be disturbed. At this point, the more you "let go" and allow your body to get on with what it knows how to do, the better.

Your needs may change rapidly during this stage – one minute you want a massage, the next you cannot bear to be touched. Your birth partner must simply BE there for you, accepting how you feel at any given moment.

You are totally absorbed and your birth partner may see a determination that he or she has not seen before as you become focused and withdrawn. Again it is important to stress that you do not make the mistake of going to hospital too soon. This stage can last for four to eight hours. One tip for the birth partner is to take your picture just as you are getting ready to go to hospital – if you are still smiling then you are not yet ready to go! If that is the case, stay at home a bit longer.

This is the time to really get primal, and to create a quiet, dark, warm and safe environment – the more you can birth like a mammal, the better.

So, when should you make the move if you are not planning a home birth?

Obviously, this will depend on how far you have to go, the time of day, the weather and traffic. However, here are a few key milestones in the birth journey which your birth partner should look out for:

- Your contractions are 60–90 seconds and coming every 3 minutes.

- Your face is continually flushed.

- You have any shaking, vomiting or hiccups.

Life is always a rich and steady time when you are waiting for something to happen or to hatch – E. B. White, "Charlotte's Web"

- You have another bloody show.

- If you feel any rectal pressure or the urge to push, go immediately, or call an ambulance or your midwife and prepare to stay at home.

- You have the instinct that now is the time to go in.

Phase 3. Self-doubt phase

This is often the most mismanaged part of labour. Unlike the other two phases, which can go on for long periods of time, the self-doubt usually comes in short bursts, often a couple of times during the later stages of labour.

If you and your birth partner do not know about it, then it can often lead to unnecessary action being taken, such as either of you asking the medical team to "do something" to help. Having the awareness that this is a normal part of labour and an indication that you are progressing really well or that you are close to having your baby can be very reassuring, no matter what you are actually saying.

Once your labour is really well established and your body has been gradually opening up for some time, the uterus saves a burst of energy until the last few centimetres for the cervix to open. During this phase, around 7–10 cm, the uterus shifts into a higher gear and contractions become more intense and overpowering. Contractions may be 60–90 seconds long and about 2 minutes apart.

Self-doubt is as it says – a time when you suddenly feel that you are unsure that you will be able to carry on. This usually occurs towards the end of labour and can happen a couple of times. The first can be when you are in serious labour, when your body is moving to the next level (often around 7 cm if we have to put a number on it) and then again when your body is almost ready to begin pushing out your baby.

You may become more outwardly focused and can experience this sense of self-doubt over whether you can go on much longer. You may wonder why it is taking so long and why the baby is not coming, thinking things like, "I don't think I can go on much longer", "I want to go home", "Get this baby out of me", and so on. However, externally you may appear to be coping really well.

If we make our goal to live a life of compassion and unconditional love, then the world will indeed become a garden where all kinds of flowers can bloom and grow –
Daphne Rose Kingma

Your body may also be showing physical signs that your body is working really hard – hot and cold flushes, shaking, nausea and vomiting. These are normal physical responses to hard work – just as, when you have run a marathon or carried a heavy object a long way, you can feel hot and shaky or a little nauseous. However, it is useful for you and your birth partner to know about them so that you are not surprised or shocked if they happen.

This is the time to really relax, really ride with it and take each contraction for what it is, and focus only on the present moment (see step 2 later in the book). Your birth partner needs to listen attentively to your breathing. You may now have to control the speed of breathing, slow it down, and really concentrate on a super-limp body.

Remember, at all times, that you are simply experiencing a feeling – a sensation within your body that you can work with. The most important thing is for you to accept the powerful sensations – they cannot "overpower you" because they are part of you, working to give birth to your baby. It is intense, hard, and challenging, but can also be incredible and truly awesome.

This is the time for your supporters to really encourage you, really praise you. To let you know that you are soon going to give birth to your baby, that you are so close to the end, that everything is normal and that you and your baby are OK and doing what nature intended.

If your birth partner is unaware that this self-doubt is normal and to be expected, it is often the most blundered and badly handled part of birth, as your partner is more likely to seek additional assistance on your behalf.

So it is THE TIME TO WAIT, FOCUS AND HOLD OFF ANY INTERVENTION.

Your partner needs to remind you that you have done so well up until now and that you have only a short time to go. Once you feel that urge to push your baby out, then all the self-doubt will go and you will become more energised and determined.

Having explored the physical, hormonal and emotional map of birth, I hope you can see how giving birth is so exquisitely designed and how a woman's body, when she is left alone to birth her baby instinctively, knows exactly what to do.

It is this instinctive model of birthing that will now stay at the forefront of your mind so that all your actions and thoughts will set you up mentally and emotionally to follow that path.

Love cures people – both the ones who give it and the ones who receive it
– Karl A. Menninger

With that in mind, it is a useful exercise to explore why and how fear and anxiety have become such a prevalent and negative part of other women's birth experiences in the westernised world.

That way, you can take active steps to avoid that happening when you go into labour.

---

[1] Gaskin, Ina May, 2003, *Ina May's Guide to Childbirth*, Bantam Dell.

[2] Bloom, S. L., Casey, B. M., Schaffer, J. I., McIntire, D. D., & Leveno, K. J., 2006, A Randomised Trial of Coached versus Uncoached Maternal Pushing During the Second Stage of Labor. *American Journal of Obstetrics and   Gynaecology,* 194, 10–13.

[3] Gaskin, Ina May, 2003, *Ina May's Guide to Childbirth*, Bantam Dell.

[4] Odent, M., 2003, *Primal Health*, Clairview.

[5] Ainsworth, S., 2005, *Quick Start, Practicing Midwife*, 8(5) p. 58.

[6] Odent, M., 1999, *The Scientification of Love*, London Free Press.

[7] Odent, M., 1999, *The Scientification of Love*, London Free Press.

[8] Kuchinskas, J. (2008), Mitzi (2005).

[9] Anderson, T., 2000, Feeling Safe Enough to Let Go, chapter 5 in Kirkham, M. (ed), 2000, *The Midwife-Mother Relationship*, Hampshire: Palgrave Macmillan.

[10] Ray Mears, 2005, *Survival*, BBC.

[11] Odent, M., 1999, *The Scientification of Love*, London Free Press.

A mother's love liberates – Maya Angelou

A dad's experience

"One of the things that stuck in my mind from the course was the 'self-doubt' phase. I had never heard about it and yet it made complete sense.

On the day, I was so pleased I knew about this, as I was able to manage it in a completely different way than I would have done. We had planned a home birth and so the first time she went through self-doubt was when she suddenly said she needed an epidural. She had been so dead against this that I felt sure she was in self-doubt. I suggested that we have three more contractions and then make a decision.

She reluctantly agreed, and during those contractions I reminded her of things that she had done in the past when she wanted to give up, but then found the strength to carry on – for example, when we went walking in the foothills of the Himalayas, she had sat down on the mountain path and refused to move. She did of course manage to carry on. We also did shaking the apples [see step 4] and '3, 2, 1, relax'; within fifteen minutes she was back on track and did not ask for the epidural again.

The second time was when she was in the pool and again suddenly said she had had enough and could not do any more. I smiled to myself as I knew that this was the self-doubt phase again, so I said how well she was doing and that this was a sign that our baby was soon going to be born. Sure enough, she started to push a few minutes later.

Thank you so much for teaching us this, as without it I would definitely have hit the panic button and things would have turned out very differently."

Bill Baines, South Africa

A mum's experience

"Things started off slowly with a mild backache and an ache under my bump that generally lasted for about 20 to 30 seconds. It was not too much of a bother, though. I kept repeating '3, 2, 1, relax', and I was able to put up with it. At about 9 a.m. I woke David and told him that I was feeling some discomfort. He asked me if it was labour, but I honestly did not know, so we decided to get on with our day.

Within an hour David was sure that I was in labour, so he called the hospital to let them know. We felt very much in the excitement phase, so we walked to the local high street and went to the post office, the library and a coffee shop. By midday we went back home and I had a bath. David helped me to continue to use the Natal Hypnotherapy techniques that we had learned.

At 4 p.m. David had to persuade me to go to the hospital, as I was sure that it was too soon and that we would just be sent home. David recognised this as part of the self-doubt phase and cajoled me into the car. At the hospital I was asked if they could give me a quick exam. David and I were happy for this. As I climbed onto the bed my waters broke. There was meconium in my waters, so the midwife asked if she could monitor the baby. She also asked if I would like any pain relief, so I opted for the gas and air. I was not feeling overly sociable, so, after David asked the reason for monitoring, we agreed to it.

The midwife was very helpful. She said that I was 8 cm dilated and that the part that was left to dilate was all on one side. She then suggested a position that would assist. A few contractions later and I was fully dilated. It was then just a matter of pushing. Our baby girl was born at 7 p.m., weighing 8 lbs 5 oz.

The Natal Hypnotherapy techniques were incredibly helpful to me during the labour, allowing me to achieve a fairly natural birth (gas aside). David found the gatekeeper role and emotional map of labour to be invaluable in helping him assess what stage in the process we were at and what needed to be done. We are both hugely grateful for everything that we learned from the course. It had a really positive impact on us and enabled us to have the sort of birth experience that we wanted."

Samantha Jones, UK

Chapter 3 – The history of a fear-based birth culture

As you can now see, when a woman gives birth in a supportive environment with the right conditions, birth can be an amazing, instinctive and powerful experience. Sadly, this is far removed from the classic media portrayal of women screaming in terror and agony.

So why is there such a discrepancy? Why do most women not talk about birth the way it has just been described? Well, you probably already know the answer.

Over stimulation of the intellectual part of the brain (the neocortex) can cause the human mind to "interfere" with the instinctive birthing process and thus lose the ability to completely let go and surrender to the mammalistic, birthing brain. The most prominent and important difference between mammals and humans is the ability to use words, to analyse and to intellectualise. Through talking about birth, hearing others' stories, reading all the things that can go wrong, watching media portrayals of birth, and so on, many women have developed particularly strong emotions of fear and anxiety towards giving birth. As we have already touched on, fear and anxiety (which are of course present in all mammals) can have a real physical impact on the progress of labour.

A study on the expectations of pain in childbirth by Green in 1993 looked at over 700 women. The results showed that:

> Anxiety about the pain of labour was a strong predictor of negative experiences during labour, lack of satisfaction with the birth and poor emotional well-being postnatally. Women tended to experience what they expected to, whether that was a lot of pain or a little.[1]

So it would seem that fear and expectations of pain are the underlying cause of much of the trauma and excessive pain in childbirth. And yet we know that birth can be instinctive, manageable, and, for some, even enjoyable.

Babies are such a nice way to start people – Don Herold

So, the next question to explore is: why is there so much fear in modern birthing, and where does it stem from?

Before we go on to look at the impact that these emotions can have on the birthing process, it is useful and interesting to have a look back in time to understand how women and society have changed from viewing birth as an empowering, enlightening, powerful and natural event, to one of which over 86% of women in the UK are terrified [2].

History of modern birth culture

If the process of giving birth is as straightforward and instinctive as described so far in this book, why are there so many perceived risks and horror stories about giving birth?

If the old phrase, "It can't be that bad, as women have done this for thousands of years" is true, then why are we seeing more and more intervention and more and more fear surrounding birth?

As one of the first pioneers to reclaim instinctive birth, Grantly Dick-Read wrote in his groundbreaking book *Childbirth without Fear*:

> the more civilized the people, the more the pain of labour appears to be intensified … the more cultured the races of the earth have become, so much the more positive they have been in promoting childbirth to be a painful and dangerous ordeal.[3]

To understand the drivers of change, it is useful to look at a short history of birth culture in Europe and then later in the US over the last 400 years. That may seem like a long time, but in fact it is just a very small chunk of time in the big scheme of things, considering that humans have been giving birth for around 200,000 years!

By understanding how perceptions and beliefs surrounding birth have changed, and by understanding how fear has become so associated with birth, you will begin to be able to untangle your own fears and beliefs connected with the birth of your baby.

As you understand how deeply and how widely the fear has permeated our birth culture, you will realise that it is a collective belief in society rather than an absolute or given truth –

Children are a handful sometimes but a heart full all the time – Author unknown just because the events of history have changed this perception of birth, that does not mean that you have to carry on the burden of fear.

It will become evident in the next chapter how detrimental this fear is to the birthing process, and how so much of the excessive pain experienced by so many women during childbirth can be attributed to the impact that fear can have on the birthing female.

Strong, healthy, instinctive women

Much of our knowledge about what birth was like in the past comes from traditional birth art as well as historical documentation from early civilisations and then later from early explorers who studied "primitive" women giving birth.

Examples of birth art and birth sculptures go back thousands of years, from Stone Age sculptures to statues in ancient Greece, from engravings from Peru to birth art from American Indians. The majority of them depict similar scenes, with women in upright positions being supported by other women. In most of this birth art, the birthing women are portrayed as serene, strong and powerful.

Anthropologists Sjoo and Mor point out that millions of years of mammalian survival can be attributed to the females physical strength, noting that:

The human race could not have survived if women had been as physically weak and mentally dependent during those hard ages as we are supposed to be today.[4]

Many birth case studies have been documented by early explorers. For example, in 1701, a traveller among the Guiana women in South America noted:

When, on the march, an Indian is taken with labour, she just steps aside, delivers and wraps up the baby with the afterbirth and runs in haste after the others.[5]

Did you know?

Traditionally, one of the most common positions for women to give birth in is kneeling up and resting their body against a tree or stool. This was referred to in the Bible, by Roman poets and in birth art from Native Americans.

People who say they sleep like a baby usually don't have one – Leo J. Burke

Complications were rare – in 1641 it was documented that:

> Women are rarely sick from childbirth, suffer no inconveniences from the same, nor do any die on such occasions.[6]

Women who gave birth using just their instincts and ancient birth knowledge were traditionally strong, fit and healthy. They continued to be active throughout pregnancy. It is interesting to note that there were no customs which prescribed that women should be careful, should slow down or restrict activity during pregnancy; in fact, it was quite the opposite – women often carried out daily physical activities right up until the birth.

By keeping active, strong and fit, they routinely used their bodies and muscles in ways which were helpful later on in childbirth. They spent much of their time squatting so that their perineal, vaginal and thigh muscles were strong and supple and they were able to give birth in positions which were instinctive and conducive to the work of the uterine muscles, and of course to gravity[7].

Did you know?

The Sanpoil tribe encourage pregnant women to remain strong and fit during their pregnancy. Women follow a regular programme of exercise, mainly of walking and swimming.

Women had healthy diets and trusted conventional wisdom about foods to avoid during pregnancy. For example, many cultures prohibited sugar; the Akamba of Kenya believed that if a mother ate sugarcane or honey, the child would become so large that a successful labour would be almost impossible[8]. In other areas, dairy produce was restricted, as were meat and spices – many cultures encouraged a vegetarian diet during pregnancy. However, what is important to remember is that since time began, women on all kinds of different diets have consistently had healthy pregnancies and given birth to strong, fit babies – whether the mothers were on a fish-only diet, such as Inuit women, or a vegetarian diet, such as women in southern India.

Traditionally, birth was in or near the home, often supported by members of a small, close-knit community, although it was also common for women to take themselves away from the group to give birth alone. During their pregnancy, women were supported by other women they knew and trusted; however, it was always the birthing woman that "birthed" her baby – she did not have her baby "delivered" by some specialised practitioner. In some cultures, women had special places to give birth in, such as the Baobab tree for the Hadza tribe in Tanzania, or purpose-built "nesting houses" for the Maori. What is consistent, though, is that women always gave birth in an environment with which they were familiar, and in which they felt safe.

Every baby needs a lap – Henry Robin

An interesting depiction of the importance of being fit, healthy and not fearing childbirth is shown in the Bible, which tells of the time before the exodus from Egypt, when all new baby boys were ordered to be killed at birth. The midwives were able to say that this could not be done, as they usually did not get there in time. These fast and easy labours were due to the Hebrew women being stronger and healthier compared to Egyptian women, who were lazy, unhealthy and unfit, and so consequently had much harder labours.

And the midwives said unto Pharaoh, Because the Hebrew women are not as the Egyptian women; for they are lively, and are delivered ere the midwives come in unto them.[9]

The tide begins to change

As Europe began to develop and move away from the agrarian, hunter-gatherer lifestyle, communities became larger and ultimately urbanisation took the place of agrarian lifestyles. This brought with it a great many changes, which contributed to a dramatic shift in the health and well-being of women and hence birthing culture. This urban crowding brought with it a poorer quality of life, increasing malnutrition, fast spread of disease, lack of sunlight and exercise, and unhygienic conditions. In these conditions, women were no longer as fit, strong and healthy, and so childbirth brought with it a whole array of complications, which in turn led to a growing fear of the consequences of childbirth.

Advent of medicine

During the Middle Ages and the Renaissance period (the thirteenth to the seventeenth century), the early development of medicine and the rise in Christianity had a profound and long-lasting impact on birth culture.

A person soon learns how little he knows when a child begins to ask questions
– Richard L. Evans

As the medical and Christian professions were only open to men, this era saw the biggest change ever seen to the culture of birth – the shift from women-centred birthing to a male-dominated medical approach.

From the fifteenth to the seventeenth century, many countries forbade women from practising medicine or religion (often closely linked). It was a time of great wariness of anything which did not strictly adhere to the rules and regulations of the Church. During this time, the women who understood how the body worked and used herbs and traditional methods to help women during labour, i.e. who were midwives or healers, were seen as heretics or witches and were executed on mass.

> In the midst of the atmosphere of change brought about by the issuance of the official mandates, determining who should administer to the sick … one of the saddest events in the history of women and healing began. The great witch hunt. It was inordinately successful in eliminating women's influence on the healing arts up to the present day. It was estimated that anywhere from a few hundred thousand to nine million women were murdered between the years 1500 and 1650.[10]

With the execution of these wise women went much of the traditional birth wisdom.

During this time, the medical profession was also developing, and of course women were banned from studying or being recognised as professionals in any way. To help with the development of medical learning, hospitals and asylums were set up as institutions to give medical students a place to learn and practise their trade.

However, they were very different places to the hospitals we know today. They were filthy, noisy, crowded places, rife with infection and disease – not a good place for a birthing woman!

However, many women, especially poor women, began to go to hospitals to have their babies, as they did not have the support of traditional midwives in their community. In addition, these institutions were often better places than their own homes and there was a growing belief that "medical" men would be able to help them. However, as hospitals were extremely dirty and there was a serious lack of hygiene, the complications and death rates in hospitals, especially from childbed fever, were extremely high.

It was only in 1847 that a wise man called Dr. Semmelweiss realised that the cause of childbed fever was the lack of hygiene amongst doctors – it was common for them to go straight from dissecting dead bodies to performing internal examinations on birthing women

It was the tiniest thing I ever decided to put my whole life into   – Terri Guillemets

without washing their hands! In one year, the death rate in his wards fell from an astounding 18 per cent to 3 per cent, and then soon after fell further to 1 per cent. It was also in 1854 that Florence Nightingale made it more widely known that cleanliness and fresh air were fundamental necessities of nursing.

It was only once it became standard practice in the 1890's for doctors in hospitals to wash their hands between patients that the maternal death rate went down. But, by that point, many generations of women had gone into labour feeling petrified of birth, knowing that death was not an unusual outcome for women going into labour.

In addition, during this time, women were no longer encouraged to be upright but were expected to lie flat on their back during labour, as it was a more convenient position for the doctor to assess how the labour was progressing. The invention of forceps in the seventeenth century ensured that women stayed flat on their back, even though traditional birth knowledge is explicitly clear on the fact that lying flat on your back is the worst-possible position for a labouring woman.

The thoughts and beliefs associated with the prevailing religious teachings played a significant part in altering the birth culture. As the male-dominated religion grew in power and popularity, the perception of women, sexual intercourse and giving birth changed significantly.

The role of women was systematically degraded and any sexual act was perceived as the ultimate sin. It became the common belief that birth was the result of the ultimate sin, for which women should pay the price. There is a famous passage in the Bible known as "the curse of Eve", in which:

> The Lord God said to Eve – I will greatly multiply thy sorrow and thy conception; in sorrow thou shalt bring forth children.[11]

Grantly Dick-Read was interested in the translation of the Bible from Hebrew to Latin, and noted that the Hebrew word "etzev" – meaning labour, toil or hard work – was mistranslated as the word "pain" when associated with childbirth (there are sixteen other uses of the word "etzev" in the Bible with the correct translation of the word). Translators had made the assumption that birth should be painful and so used the word "pain" instead of "labour" or "toil"[12].

As more and more women gave birth without the traditional love, support and birth knowledge from other women, and there were increasing numbers of complications and

Your job as a parent is to give your kids not only the instincts and talents to survive, but help them enjoy their lives – Susan Sarandon

deaths during or just after childbirth, it is not difficult to understand how women became terrified of birth.

Industrialisation of birth

By the nineteenth century, most women viewed labour as terrifyingly painful and dangerous, so when the drug chloroform was introduced, it was heralded as a major breakthrough in helping women deal with the pain of birth. When Queen Victoria was given chloroform by Dr. John Snow on 7 April 1853 for the birth of Prince Leopold, it was met with two extreme opinions. For many women, it became acceptable and then fashionable to use chloroform during labour. In fact, it was said that "her greatest gift to her people was a refusal to accept pain in childbirth as women's divinely appointed destiny"[13]. However, ministers of the Church condemned the doctor, saying that chloroform was a

> decoy of Satan, apparently offering itself to bless women; but in the end
> it will harden society and rob God of the deep earnest cries of a woman
> in childbirth.[14]

Women who had chloroform were literally knocked out during the birth and would take several days to recover from the effects of the gas. As a result, their babies were cared for by nurses in rooms which became known as nurseries. For the first time since human civilisation began, babies were routinely taken away from their mothers during a time which we now know (although traditional birth wisdom has always known!) is so crucial to the health and well-being of both mother and baby, and to the bonding between them.

So, from the 1900's onwards, yes, hospitals became cleaner; yes, giving birth was getting safer; and, yes, chloroform took all the pain away, but by then birth was so far removed from the instinctive natural process that the so-called industrialisation of birth had begun.

Natural, instinctive birthing had been replaced with processes, procedures and instruments to "control" and manage the birth, many of which are still used today. Women were routinely given enemas, dressed in hospital gowns, had their pubic hair shaved (due to a belief that lice would bring infection) and were instructed to lie flat on their backs in order to have their baby "delivered" by the doctor. Women became completely disempowered and no longer trusted their natural instincts.

Birth had become a medical event which needed to be managed by medical professionals.

The child supplies the power but the parents have to do the steering
— Benjamin Spock

And, so, as women entered the twentieth century, what was once seen as a natural part of life's cycle became something to be terrified of. A woman gave birth on her own, in a sterile, foreign environment, surrounded by strange men and women. In the back of her mind were all the stories she had heard about agonising pain and possible death. She was told what to do and where to go, and accepted any intervention that she was subjected to without question.

She felt alone, scared, passive and disempowered. She was then drugged up to the eyeballs, feeling completely out of control, often strapped to a bed and routinely cut while her baby was dragged out of her using forceps. She was then so doped-up that she could not even hold or take care of her baby, let alone breastfeed, for several days after the birth.

Is it any wonder that women became so fearful of giving birth?

This is a very gloomy and upsetting picture; however, it has been written for a reason. Now that you understand where modern birth culture has come from, it will become easier to recognise where many women's fears stem from. The most important thing to remember from this is that although times have changed and the world around us has moved on, the woman's body and the inbuilt process of birthing, which has been there for thousands and thousnds of years, has not!

Modern antenatal care

Luckily, the picture of modern birthing today is quite different from the one at the turn of the last century, and many wonderful steps have been taken to address the issues and to turn the corner towards making birth more natural and instinctive.

However, there are still too many procedures taking place which interfere with a woman's instincts and the natural flow of pregnancy and birth, and which often introduce unacceptably high levels of fear and anxiety and intervention (see chapter on 'Maternity guidelines – It's your choice').

Think back to the beginning of your pregnancy.

- Did you trust in your instincts?
- Did you know that you were pregnant?
- Did you feel the need to wee on a stick to get external confirmation that you really were pregnant?

The world talks to the mind. Parents speak more intimately – they talk to the heart
– Haim Ginott

In our society today, from the moment a woman becomes pregnant, she relies on external factors to tell her everything is OK. Many women no longer know how to trust their body – from the earliest time, a woman will seek external "affirmation" that she is pregnant by using a pregnancy test.

Women no longer rely on the age-old changes in their body to let them know they are pregnant. And then, from the moment they realise that they are pregnant, many women begin worrying about what they are consuming. Have they had any wine? Have they had any unpasteurised products? Have they taken any paracetamol? Have they taken enough folic acid?

Women are bombarded with all the things that could damage the foetus, all the things they MUST not do: what to eat, what not to eat, how to sleep, how to exercise and so on, which often seems more pointless when the "rules" are so different from one country to another.

From the first appointment with a birth professional, a woman is essentially treated as high risk; in other words, she needs to take a whole series of tests to "prove" that everything is OK – blood tests, urine tests, blood pressure monitored, etc. So, from the very first appointment, there is an element of anxiety. What if the tests come back negative? What if the blood pressure is too high? Even after twelve weeks, many women do not really trust their bodies, or believe that they are pregnant, until they see their baby on a screen at their first scan.

Even though pregnancy is the most normal, natural event, and one which has happened every day for millennia, we have taken the "what if" scenario to it's extreme. Many women spend the next several months reading pregnancy magazines ("I gave birth on the motorway", "My Caesarean nightmare", "How Group Strep B nearly killed me"), searching the Internet and watching Discovery Health, seeking out all pregnancy and birth-related information – for good and bad.

And what does all that do to a woman's emotional and mental state? Quite often it simply increases her levels of anxiety and fear about all the things that could go wrong.

Even though being pregnant and giving birth is not a medical procedure, it is ironic that there is no other medical procedure in which the "patient" is given so much information and told in such great detail what will happen. If you are having a tooth out or your tonsils out, would you know the name of the drugs given as pain relief or the names of the instruments used? No – you accept that the medical professionals know what they are doing and will use the appropriate equipment when necessary.

And yet there is plenty of clinical evidence to show that all the "routine" procedures – such as regular blood-pressure tests[15], routine scans[16] and even continual foetal monitoring[17] during

There are two lasting bequests we can give our children. One is roots. The other is wings – Hodding Carter, Jr.

labour – do not actually produce better outcomes for mum or baby. In fact, as Michel Odent argues, over-the-top routine antenatal care produces a "nocebo" effect (the opposite of placebo), creating more harm from the belief that things can go wrong.

> The nocebo effect is a negative effect on the emotional state of pregnant women and indirectly of their families. It occurs whenever a health professional makes more harm than good by interfering with the imagination, the fantasy life or the beliefs of a patient or a pregnant woman.[18]

Many women feel that they are preparing for birth by learning as much as they can about all the procedures and guidelines, and by knowing all the relevant risks and possible dangers. Many antenatal classes spend more time talking about which drugs will be available, what the hospital procedures are and which instruments will be used than they do about helping a woman to feel more confident and trusting in what is essentially an instinctive event.

This kind of preparation is appealing to our human intellect, our need to be in control; but, unfortunately, this type of knowledge can often exacerbate the problem, as it can lead to increased levels of anxiety and fear. As Pam England so nicely puts it:

> Understanding birth technology shouldn't lull you into thinking you understand birth.[19]

As we will see later, all this knowledge can then prevent the primitive part of the brain and the body's birthing muscles from working as effectively as they can, thus, ironically, leading to the need for medical intervention to "move things along" or speed things up (more on that later).

Sadly, in spite of the increase in antenatal classes, there is no evidence to suggest that this type of preparation has led to couples feeling any less anxious or fearful or led to improved birth outcomes. In addition, the rate of intervention over the last thirty years has dramatically increased, and more and more women feel traumatised, out of control, and scared of birth, with 86% of women being terrified of birth.[20]

It is important to stress that I do not believe that this has anything to do with the well-intentioned, passionate and dedicated work of birth professionals, or that women should not be informed. The problem is that women are not routinely being given the emotional and psychological support to help them prepare for birth.

> *There are three reasons for breastfeeding: the milk is always at the right temperature; it comes in attractive containers; and the cat can't get it – Irena Chalmers*

I believe that, as all the learning in antenatal classes is done in the conscious, rational, analytical part of the mind, it does not adequately address the individual's beliefs, emotions, fears or concerns. Therefore, no matter how much "intellectual learning" is done, without addressing these fundamental issues, women are not adequately prepared for birth.

As you read earlier, generations of women have gone into labour feeling and being frightened and scared. In our culture of highly medicalised births, the commonly accepted belief is that birth is excruciatingly painful and can be very traumatic, and that women need technical equipment and medical professionals to help them birth their babies.

This deeply held belief is fuelled by the media portrayal of birth, including hospital dramas, birth scenes in soaps or films and the plethora of birth-related documentaries – the majority of which focus on highly medicalised hospital environments, in which the woman is essentially a patient and under the control of the medical professionals who are seen to be her saviours and are there to "deliver" her baby.

Again, based on this fear and belief that we need medical technology to safely birth our babies, the majority of women in the western world today choose to have their babies in hospital.

However, it might be useful to stop for a moment and think about hospitals.

How do they make you feel?

What emotions does a hospital usually represent?

How do you feel about the smells, colours and sounds?

Why do most people go into hospital?

In general, hospitals are places to go when you are ill. When you go into hospital, you are there to be treated, to be a patient, to benefit from the knowledge and experience of the medical profession, whose sole purpose is to help you get better. In our modern world, we are extremely lucky that we have such medically advanced and technically superior hospitals, which save lives and help the sick get better. When needed, hospitals are a odsend.

Did you know?

Research has shown that it is as safe, if not safer, for a healthy pregnant woman to give birth at her own home attended by community midwives as it is in hospital.

Women do not have to sacrifice personhood if they are mothers. They do not have to sacrifice motherhood in order to be persons – Elaine Heffner

And yet we all know that the environment, the sights, the smells and the sounds can be intimidating and anxiety ridden. Many people become passive and hand control over to the medical staff, believing and feeling that they must know best. 'White coat syndrome' kicks in, often leading to patients feeling vulnerable, lacking in confidence and feeling the need to "do what they are told".

Instinct goes out the window and is replaced by subservience and faith in the medical care given by those around you.

So you can see how, often, all of these factors come into play when a healthy, "normal" woman goes into hospital to have her baby. Women have been led to believe that they need to be there "just in case" something goes wrong. So, at a conscious, and more importantly at a subconscious, level, simply going into hospital when a woman is in labour has the effect of diminishing her confidence, belief and sense of trust in her ability to give birth, and often dramatically increases her levels of anxiety and fear.

It is worth adding at this point that it has been shown that, for a healthy woman who has had a healthy pregnancy, giving birth at home is as safe, if not safer, than giving birth in hospital[21].

Remember back to earlier, when you read about how women have given birth since time began – choosing a place that is familiar, safe, and surrounded by people they know, or choosing somewhere close by that is safe and private.

Think about the cat that gives birth, choosing to go into a cupboard or under the bed – a warm, dark, safe, private place. By removing any external distractions, giving birth becomes more instinctive and so often easier and smoother.

You may be thinking that that is all fine for others, but you still want to go into hospital.

The most important thing is that the place you choose to give birth in is the place in which you feel the safest. If that is a hospital for you, then the crucial next steps are to help yourself use the environment to positive effect and to increase your inherent trust and belief that you can birth your baby – no matter where that is.

The secrets to having a positive birth experience in the modern technological environment are:

- To reconnect with your natural birthing instinct

A baby is an inestimable blessing and bother – Mark Twain

- To allow yourself to trust that your body is perfectly designed to birth your baby when unhindered by processes and drugs

- To prepare yourself mentally to hand control over to the primal birthing part of your body

- To learn techniques to help you keep your levels of fear and anxiety to a minimum

Did you know?

In spite of the industrialisation of birth in the modern world, **90% of everyone alive in the world today was born at home.**

The fear-based birthing culture will only begin to change if women take responsibility for their own birth experiences and become aware of the power that they have within themselves.

[1] Green, J. M., "Expectations and Experiences of Pain in Labour: Findings from a Large Prospective Study". This paper was presented at the Tenth Birth Conference, "Innovations in Prenatal Care: Assessing Benefits and Risks", October 31–November 1, 1992, Boston.

[2] *Mother and Baby* magazine survey, 2000.

[3] Dick-Read, G., 2003, *Childbirth without Fear*, Pinter & Martin.

[4] Sjoo, Monica and Mor, Barbara, 1987, *The Great Cosmic Mother*, p. 84, New York: Harper and Roa.

[5] George J. Englemann, *Labour among Primitive Peoples* (St Louis MO:JH chambers 1882: reprint New York AMS press).

[6] Adriaen Van Der Donck, 1656, *A Description of the New Netherlands*.

[7] George J. Englemann, *Labour among Primitive Peoples* (St Louis MO:JH chambers 1882: reprint New York AMS press).

[8] Gerhard Lindblom, 1916, *The Akamba in British East Africa*, Sweden, Uppsala.

[9] *The Bible*, Book of Moses Exodus. Chp 1 verse 19.

[10] Jeanne Achterberg, 1985, *Imagery in Healing*.

[11] Genesis, third chapter, verse 16.

[12] Rev B. D. Glass, Grantly Dick-Read, 2003, *Childbirth without Fear*, Pinter & Martin, p. 88.

[13] Wohl, Anthony S., 1978, *The Victorian Family, Structure and Stresses*, Croom Helm Ltd, p. 25.

[14] Wohl, Anthony S., 1978, *The Victorian Family, Structure and Stresses*, Croom Helm Ltd, p. 25.

The family you come from isn't as important as the family you're going to have
– Ring Lardner

[15] Symonds, E. M. "Aetiology of pre-eclampsia: a review". J R Soc Med 1980; 73: 871–75.
Naoyo E. M. "Maternal blood pressure and fetal growth" Am J Obstet Gynecol 1981; 141: 780–87.
Kilpatrick S. "Unlike pre-eclampsia, gestational hypertension is not associated with increased neonatal and maternal morbidity except abruptio". SPO abstracts. Am J Obstet Gynecol 1995; 419: 376. Curtis S., et al. "Pregnancy effects of non-proteinuric gestational hypertension". SPO Abstracts. Am J Obst Gynecol 1995; 418: 376.

[16] Larson T., Falck Larson J., et al. "Detection of small-for-gestational-age fetuses by ultrasound screening in a high risk population: a randomized controlled study". Br J Obstet Gynaecol 1992; 99: 469–74. Secher N. J., Kern Hansen P., et al. "A randomized study of fetal abdominal diameter and fetal weight estimation for detection of light-for-gestation infants in low-risk pregnancy". Br J Obstet Gynaecol 1987; 94: 105–9.

[17] Thacker S. B., Stroup D. F. "Continuous electronic heart rate monitoring versus intermittent auscultation for assessment during labor". Cochrane Database Syst Rev 1999 (Issue No. 3).

[18] Odent M. "The Nocebo effect in prenatal care". Primal Health Research Newsletter 1994; 2 (2). Odent M. "Back to the Nocebo effect". Primal Health Research Newsletter 1995; 5 (4). Odent M. "Antenatal scare". Primal Health Research Newsletter 2000; 7 (4).

[19] England, Pam, 2007, *Birth from Within*, England & Horowitz.

[20] *Mother and Baby* magazine survey, 2000.

[21] Janssen P. A., Lee S. K., Ryan E. M., Etches D. J., Farquharson D. F., Peacock D., Klein M. C. "Outcomes of planned home births versus planned hospital births after regulation of midwifery in British Columbia", Centre for Community Health and Health Evaluation Research, BC Research Institute for Children's and Women's Health, Vancouver. pjanssen@interchange.ubc.ca
http://www.nhs.uk/news/2009/04April/Pages/HomeBirthSafe.aspx.

Nothing contributes so much to tranquillise the mind as a steady purpose – a point on which the soul may fix its intellectual eye – Mary Shelley

A mum's experience

"I became interested in using hypnotherapy to prepare for my little boy's birth because I have had a seriously deep fear of giving birth ever since I can remember. As a little girl I always said that I would never have children, and this was further compounded by the experiences of the women in my family. When I was eighteen my mum found out she was pregnant, and I was present at my brother's birth. Without going into details, my mum and I were both severely traumatised by the birth.

My sister had a similarly traumatic birth and needed reconstructive surgery. The care they both received from the midwives they encountered was appalling – from being told not to 'crap on the bed' to being left unconscious on a corridor floor after losing large amounts of blood.

Years later I met my husband and we decided to try for a baby. It took many years for us to conceive and when we finally did we were ecstatic. Unfortunately, I suffered a miscarriage at 9/10 weeks, which was devastating for us both. However, four months later I found out I was pregnant again with our little one, Isaac. The first few months were incredibly difficult, as I was in a lot of pain and bled heavily. We were terrified we might lose this pregnancy too.

My fears of giving birth resurfaced and I thought the only way I could possibly cope would be to have a C-section. At that point, I truly felt that a C-section was the only way I could gain some control over the whole process. I had watched my mum and sister go into hospital and almost cease to exist. The medical professionals had performed procedures and interventions on them, and my mum and sister had been totally passive and excluded from the decision-making processes.

Once I accepted that I wouldn't be given a C-section on the NHS and that we couldn't afford to pay for one, my next hope was that I could have an epidural so that I would be in less pain and therefore be less vulnerable and more in control. I have scoliosis, and after a consultation with the anaesthetist it became clear that this really wouldn't be an option for me, as my spine and pelvis are both twisted in a way that isn't serious, but which makes an epidural less effective and possibly completely ineffective. I felt distraught. It is difficult to explain just how terrified I felt. It went way beyond the normal trepidation that all women feel at the thought of giving birth.

I am so lucky to have found out about Natal Hypnotherapy. I began listening to the pregnancy relaxation track every day and booked a place on one of the courses. I began the course believing that I could never feel positive about giving birth and that I was not physically capable of birthing my baby without intervention; I was terrified that I would not be able to cope with the pain. I feared losing control and I feared the medical staff. During the course I slowly began to open up to the possibility that, perhaps, I might be able to trust my body, and to trust that on a deep, primal level I already knew everything I needed in order to give birth.

The lady who ran the course spoke from personal experience and was approachable and friendly yet very professional. She was able to very gently suggest that I should trust my husband more and she helped us both to fully appreciate his very important role as the 'gatekeeper'. We finished the course feeling so much closer and connected to one another. My husband had been feeling overwhelmed and powerless to help me, and I had been pushing him away. After the course, he had many practical techniques to practise with me in the run-up to the birth and had a clear idea of what his role would be. I think this helped him to feel that he was doing something useful and real to help me overcome my fears.

I practised the techniques from the course and listened to my track every day and usually more than once a day! By the end of my pregnancy I was actually looking forward to the birth with a sense of excitement and anticipation! Of course, I had a few nerves, but the major emotion I felt as my due date approached was excitement. I went into labour after some acupuncture at forty-one weeks.

I put on my music, had a bath, lit some candles and went off to my safe place. I actually enjoyed the feelings and felt waves of excitement that my baby would soon be here.

I can't really remember the following hours clearly, as my perception of time was so distorted and I was so deeply relaxed. I remember my husband telling me that we needed to go to the hospital, as my contractions had been less than a minute apart and were lasting over a minute each time. I was starting to feel them at this point too and agreed to go.

I didn't know it then, but my baby would be born two-and-a-half hours later. Once I arrived at the hospital, everything continued to go well. Even though I didn't feel able to fully relax in hospital, the hypnosis continued to work and my body simply did what it needed to do! Isaac arrived without any interventions, and without a single stitch or any pain relief (apart from a little gas and air), and I can honestly say it was the most empowering experience of my life. I birthed my baby! The midwife said that the birth was a "midwife's dream birth" and told me that when I have another baby I should consider a home birth.

Natal Hypnotherapy played such an enormous role in helping me to over-come my fears. I enjoyed my pregnancy and, yes, I would go so far as to say I enjoyed the birth too. (Although it was painful towards the end, it was manageable pain.) The course helped my husband and I to truly share the experience together. I am so proud of the journey I went on, from terror and passivity to excitement and strength – I can't thank you enough.

Hypnosis is an amazingly powerful tool and I wish every pregnant woman could have access to your course and materials. I am seriously considering training myself in the future."

Sara Allman, UK

Chapter 4 – The Impact of fear on pain

So, why and how does this fear impact your body's ability to give birth?

Remember the woman giving birth in the jungle? Fearing that there was a wild animal in her birth space would be enough for her contractions to slow down or even stop so that she could run away to a safe place. This is the classic "fight or flight" scenario which is our mechanism for self-preservation.

Or the chimpanzees that were being filmed for research – their sense of being observed enabled them to hold off contractions until the cameras had stopped rolling. The emotions of fear or anxiety have an incredibly powerful effect on a labouring female.

> Self preservation can take priority over childbirth. When a female mammal is in labour, seeing a dangerous animal will frighten her and make her secrete hormones such as adrenaline. This will interrupt the blood supply to the uterus and placenta and have the effect of sending blood rushing to the brain and muscles so that the animal can fight or run away quickly.[1]

You may be asking, "What do chimpanzees or a women giving birth in a jungle have to do with me? I have no intention of giving birth within a hundred miles of a wild animal!"

Well, one of the interesting facts about our brain is that we cannot distinguish between fear that is real, such as a tiger standing in front of us, and fear of something which is imagined, yet to happen or might happen, e.g. the potential for pain, intervention, injections, etc. No matter what the fear derives from, the physical and emotional response is the same.

For example, have you ever felt the rush of adrenalin and fear when watching a horror movie? What happens to your heartbeat, your palms, your breathing? Is the threat real or imagined? Are you really in danger from the axe murderer, or are you sitting safely in a comfortable chair at home?

Or how about waking up from a bad dream? Your mind is racing, your body is tense, and you may be sweating – real physical responses to a fear created in your mind.

If you want children to keep their feet on the ground, put some responsibility on their shoulders – Abigail Van Buren

No, we do not have wild animals near us that cause the fear; however, many women are now faced with mental and emotional fears of what might happen, which can have an equally powerful effect on their birth experience. Whether your fear comes from a birth video you saw in biology class when you were twelve, or the horror stories your friends told you, or even the stories of your own birth, that fear is real to you.

So what exactly happens in a woman's body if she is feeling frightened or anxious, and what effect will this have on her, her baby and her body's natural process of birthing?

1. Fear or anxiety will trigger the production of a hormone called adrenalin, which prepares the body for "fight or flight".

2. This leads to blood rushing away from the centre of the woman's body and being redistributed to her brain and limbs. This takes blood away from the uterus – the set of muscles that **really** need fresh oxygenated blood – and away from her baby. When the muscles of the uterus are not getting fresh oxygen, they are not as easily able to get rid of the lactic acid which is produced when muscles are working hard; lactic acid needs to be excreted, or else pain increases. The muscles therefore lose some of their elasticity (essential when flexing and releasing), becoming harder and tighter. On top of that, the baby is not getting an abundant supply of fresh oxygen through the mother's blood, and so, over a long period of time, can begin to get distressed.

3. The muscles in her body will tense up, ready to fight or run away. In a birthing woman, the most significant muscles to tense up are the circular muscles of the cervix – keeping those tight to make sure the baby CANNOT be born when a mother does not feel safe. However, the long muscles continue to stretch and flex to try and open the circular muscles. So, essentially, the cervix and the uterus are fighting against each other.

    Imagine how much harder it will be for the muscles of the uterus to open the cervix if it is all tense and refusing to budge! As all the muscles around the uterus and cervix are also tense, the poor old uterus is having to fight against the strain, rather than being free to contract and release.

A man travels the world over in search of what he needs, and returns home to find it
– George Moore

You already know how much more painful things are if you tense your muscles, for example if you are having an injection. So, is it any wonder that, with all the tension in her body, the contractions are far more painful and less productive?

4. The adrenalin neutralises the wonderful birthing hormones, including oxytocin (the one that makes the uterus contract and release), endorphins (natural painkillers), and relaxin (helps with elasticity of the muscles). The hormones, oxytocin and endorphins influence the degree to which we interpret feelings as pain or pleasure. If you reduce these hormones, then the perception of pain will go way up.

5. All this "fight or flight" preparation uses a great deal of energy. As our bodies were only designed to be in this heightened sense of being prepared to fight or flight for a few minutes at a time, you can imagine that staying in this state for prolonged periods of time will be extremely draining and possibly even harmful to the woman's baby.

   In addition, the longer she is in a state of tension, the less efficient her body becomes at flowing with the rhythm of birth.

All of the above are incredibly useful if there is a true reason to fight or run away; however, when there is no actual object of fear that can be dealt with, such as a wild animal, this state can go on indefinitely. This adrenalin-pumped situation was designed to last a few minutes. However, if it is prolonged, a woman will become exhausted, her baby can become distressed[2] and her cervix may stop opening, or even close up (see 'sphincter law').

Fear – tension – pain

"The strain in pain lies mainly in the brain."

The fear-tension-pain phrase was first coined by Grantly Dick-Read in 1942, following his study of women who gave birth and did not feel significant pain.

Fear results in tension; tension results in pain; pain leads to fear of the next contraction, and the cycle is repeated. Dick-Read believed that birth is not naturally painful and that it was culturally induced fears that played a significant part in the pain cycle.

Families are like fudge ... mostly sweet with a few nuts – Author unknown

The fear-tension-pain syndrome not only explains the origin of the discomforts of normal labour but has led to the discovery of a simple method of avoiding severe pain. By removing fear, tension and pain are minimised.[3]

He believed that removing ignorance was the key to removing fear, and teaching relaxation techniques could break the cycle and alter the perception of fear. You cannot have tension and relaxation in the body at the same time – they are opposite ends of the spectrum. Therefore, if you are relaxed, you will not have the tension, and thus you will not have the pain. He pioneered the start of antenatal classes as a way to better inform pregnant mothers.

It is easy to see how this cycle can come into play in modern birthing, as the natural and protective "fight or flight" mechanism takes place day after day in hospitals.

Imagine now that a woman is labouring beautifully at home, managing the sensations, feeling at ease being in her own surroundings, watching TV or listening to music. Then things are hotting up and it is time to go to the hospital. First of all, making sure she has everything with her, she has turned off the lights, called whom she needs to, locked the front door, gone out into the cold and got into the car. Just these alone use up valuable energy and can create a level of anxiety. She then has to sit, with a seatbelt on ... Ugh ... the worst position to be in when having a contraction. Her next thoughts may revolve around the traffic, breaking down, not getting there on time – stress ... anxiety ... aahhh – she finally gets there.

She then enters the hospital and is suddenly surrounded by strangers, and is being asked lots of questions; there are new and strange smells, noises, machines; and from now on she is

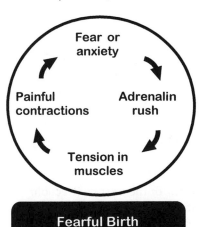

being observed. At a primal level, she is so far removed from the natural instinctive birthing environment that her levels of adrenalin have shot up and her body is attempting to try to stop or slow down labour until she feels safe and calm. As time goes by, her levels of adrenalin and anxiety reach excessive levels. By now her body is so tense that even though her uterus is still contracting, her cervix stops opening.

People around her start using terms like "oh, not dilating fast enough", "failure to progress" and "baby in distress", which leads to more anxiety, more adrenalin and usually a roller coaster of intervention to "speed things up". Once she is given any artificial hormones or chemical drugs, her body stops producing the right amount and balance of

You don't choose your family. They are God's gift to you, as you are to them
– Desmond Tutu

natural hormones, including the wonderfully powerful endorphins or natural painkillers, and so her body is struggling even more to flow through birth.

All of these factors have the ability to slow down or even stop labour, and a woman going through this truly does experience excruciating pain, which in turn reinforces the fear of the next contraction, and so the cycle goes on.

As you can see, a woman can become so entrenched in this horrible cycle that her body continues to hold back from birthing her baby, which may partly explain the current drastically high rates of chemical augmentation of labour and increase of Caesarean sections due to "failure to progress" – the most common reason for Caesarean sections today. It may also help to explain the rising rate of inductions, as the fear of birth may even prevent some women going into spontaneous labour.

It is ironic to note that the more civilised the society, the more scientific knowledge we have of the body, and the more technical advantages and medical advancements that we have made, the further we have got from the natural process designed over millions of years of evolution .... and the more birth is perceived as painful!

All the while that there is fear in childbirth, a woman's birthing body will not be allowed to flow through the natural progression of labour.

Moving on to more positive thoughts

So, enough of the negative. You are a woman giving birth in today's modern world. What active steps can you take to stay out of the fear-tension-pain cycle and help yourself give birth instinctively?

What do you need to do to find a balance between the beliefs of the woman in the story at the beginning of this book and the way many women give birth in today's world?

As we agreed, most of us do not live in a totally natural, communal environment where the birth culture is instinctive and integrated into our daily lives. Instead, we live in a society where we need to abide by certain rules and guidelines, and one in which a predominantly medical model of the world prevails. Of course, this also means that we are fortunate enough to have amazing medical care and resources available when true life-threatening emergencies occur.

If your baby is "beautiful and perfect, never cries or fusses, sleeps on schedule and burps on demand, an angel all the time", you're the grandma – Teresa Bloomingdale

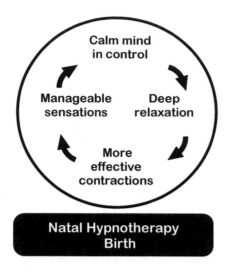

It may seem a little daunting or it may even feel wonderfully exciting, knowing that you can reconnect with your instincts, that you can overcome your fears and that you can truly trust your body, so that no matter where or how you birth your baby, it will be a fulfilling, positive and empowering experience.

So, how can you make the best of the good things around you and still ensure that you can birth your baby in a way that is instinctive and primal?

How can you break out of the fear-tension-pain cycle to one of calm and relaxation?

Read on to find out how, by following **5 simple steps**, you can move from the fear-tension-pain scenario to one of calm, relaxation, and more-effective and manageable contractions.

[1] Odent, M, 2003, *Primal Health*, Clairview.

[2] Lederman, R. P. et al., "Anxiety and epinephrine in multiparous women in labour: relationship to duration of labor and fetal heart rate pattern". *Am J Obstet Gynecol* 1985;153(8):870–7.

[3] Dick-Read, G., 2004, *Childbirth without Fear*, page 45; Pinter & Martin Ltd.

Don't limit yourself. Many people limit themselves to what they think they can do. You can go as far as your mind lets you. What you believe, remember, you can achieve
– Mary Kay Ash

A mum's experience

"My pregnancy was not easy. I suffered with pain in the beginning, with fear of an ectopic pregnancy or early miscarriage, as my hormone levels did not rise as expected. I then suffered terrible nausea for the first five months, pelvic discomfort and sciatica, and finally was diagnosed with gestational diabetes at thirty-two weeks.

I found the Natal Hypnotherapy site through the home birth website. The stories on that site were such an inspiration. I always had the belief that childbirth is a natural process that I could manage, but being an experienced nurse I knew that a hospital birth was more likely to be medicalised and I would not be in control.

I began practising Natal Hypnotherapy early on in my pregnancy and found the techniques really helpful in strengthening my belief in myself and my baby's ability to get through labour and the birth. I even began to look forward to it through the whole pregnancy. The CDs helped me to sleep, too, and I would often use them as a way to send me off into a pleasant nap during the day!

The birth preparation track was wonderful, so empowering. My husband listened to it a couple of times too while massaging my back and shoulders, so he knew the key phrases, which he used to excellent effect during the labour (we breathed a lot of golden light together!). It was a real shock being diagnosed with gestational diabetes, as I only weighed 54 kg, and ate a perfect diet throughout the pregnancy. The diabetic team advised against the home birth, but we fought hard, controlling my blood sugars perfectly with diet alone, and the baby always measured perfectly for dates.

My husband is an A&E charge nurse and a registered paediatric nurse, so we felt confident enough to manage the monitoring of my blood sugars and the baby's afterbirth, and to transfer to hospital if we were unable to keep control of them. After finally meeting with the supervisor of midwives on 26 September, we were 'allowed' our home birth. On Monday, 29 September at 6.30 p.m., my mucus plug came away. This was a surprise, as baby was not due until 17 October.

Things started to happen slowly on Tuesday, 30 September, with contractions coming every seven to ten minutes throughout the night. My midwife examined me to find that the baby was in a posterior position, meaning that the contractions were really just turning baby round to prepare for birth, and could go on for several days yet.

I managed to get some rest until the contractions woke me every four minutes. My husband put on the birth preparation track and rubbed my back through the contractions, but I knew they were doing good, as I could feel baby turning. By 1 a.m. on Thursday the contractions were every two-and-a-half minutes and very strong. I was able to keep very calm and controlled with breathing, but we decided to try the TENS for the back pains, which I found very helpful.

We had the relaxing birth music CD on from then on. I phoned the hospital at 2 a.m. to tell them I was in labour; unfortunately, there was no midwife on call to attend a home birth until 8 a.m., so I knew then that I would have to go in if things progressed. I had been so set on having a home birth and so against having to transfer to hospital during the pregnancy, but having listened to the track, I focused on the part that says wherever you are when you give birth, you will feel calm and in control, and I did.

At 3 a.m. the contractions were every two minutes, with very little time in-between, so I phoned the hospital again and they advised me to go in. Fortunately, the supervisor of midwives that I had met with to discuss my home birth was on duty, so she understood my feelings, and looked after us until 7.30 a.m., when she handed over to the next shift.

I had written a clear birth plan and handed the information-for-midwives sheet supplied with the CDs to them on our arrival. We put the birth music CD on as soon as we arrived, and the midwife checked baby's heart rate, and examined me. I was 3 cm dilated. Baby had turned, so her back was to the side. The midwife then left us alone, just checking on us every half an hour or so, and checking baby's heart rate, which stayed at 140 bpm throughout the whole labour and delivery. I tried to remain active, but my legs were like jelly; I found it really hard to stand through the contraction, so I spent most of the time leaning over the beanbag on all fours on the bed. The contractions were as the track described – strong sensations. I never perceived them as painful. In fact, the sensation of everything opening up was a pleasurable one. I can remember saying at the time that it felt nice.

At around 6 a.m. the midwife examined me again and found I was 8 cm with a lip; she suggested I sit with my back against the bed for a while, as a change of position could help. At this point, I was so tired from very little sleep for three nights that my body seemed to know it needed some rest before I could give birth, and the contractions slowed to about every five minutes. In between contractions I seemed to fall asleep instantly. I would wake for the contraction, which caused lots of involuntary spasmodic pushing, and then as it eased I would fall asleep again.

At around 8 a.m. the contractions became stronger and very frequent again. I was no longer able to sit and went back on all fours again. I then began pushing. The midwife offered me some gas and air, even though I stated in my birth plan that I did not want to be offered anything and would ask if I wanted it. The idea repulsed me.

I did not want anything to interfere with my mind and body's ability to give birth, and really didn't feel I needed it. The pushing was completely involuntary; my body knew what to do, and I just went with it. As my baby started to emerge, the midwife said the waters were still intact. I had had a small gush at the start of pushing, which must have been the hindwaters. Baby was born in her waters like a space helmet, and had a lovely round head, hardly moulded at all.

Our beautiful daughter was born at 8.58 a.m. on Thursday, 2 October. She was born with minimal assistance from the midwife in between my legs and I knelt up and picked her up and held her, skin to skin. She was so calm, she hardly cried at all. We spent some time just cuddling her. She latched on and breastfed. My husband clipped and cut the cord once it had stopped pulsating and I delivered the placenta without any injection. Around an hour later, when the midwife transferred us to the ward, she said she felt so privileged to be part of our birth. She was amazed by how calm and in control I had been and how naturally and efficiently I had pushed the baby out.

A student midwife had been present too and she came to thank us for letting her be there. She said it was so unusual to see such a calm and natural birth and it restored her faith in women's ability to give birth without any interventions. We took our daughter home that afternoon.

A few days later, when I phoned the ward, I spoke to the supervisor of midwives, who said that she had heard what a lovely birth we had had and was really impressed with the hypnotherapy. In fact, she said she was a real sceptic about it when I first told her about it but now really believed it worked. Praise indeed!

The postnatal recovery track was a real comfort through the first few weeks, and continued and consolidated the feeling of calm and control when I needed it. I am so glad I found out about Natal Hypnotherapy. We had the perfect birth; even though it was in hospital, everything happened and was done when and how we wanted it.

I recommend Natal Hypnotherapy to everyone, and feel sure my next pregnancy and birth will be as wonderful because of you.

Thank you."

Tina Davies, UK

Part 2

Chapter 5 – Natal Hypnotherapy

It has been mentioned quite a few times already, but what exactly is Natal Hypnotherapy?

Natal Hypnotherapy is a wonderful set of tools which can help you overcome fear; increase trust and confidence in your body; learn to relax deeply, breathe effectively, and stay calm no matter what is going on around you; and protect yourself from negative thoughts.

By doing all these things, you will approach birth with all you need to trust your body and to help you give birth instinctively, regardless of where you give birth to your baby.

The term Natal Hypnotherapy may be a relatively recent one; however, since time began, skilled birth attendants have used a variety of hypnotic techniques to help women stay calm and focused – chanting, dancing, belly dancing, singing, praying, and so on. Put simply, hypnotic techniques have been used as a methodical way of helping the woman focus her thoughts and shut everything else out to enable her to work with her body.

The skills and techniques of the Natal Hypnotherapy approach have been created and developed from an understanding of:

- Traditional birthing knowledge
- How the mind and body work
- What causes fear and pain in childbirth
- An understanding of the modern maternity system

Bringing all these elements together, Natal Hypnotherapy has created a new approach to birth preparation which is safe, easy to use, works in the current maternity system, and puts women back in control; and, fundamentally, the approach can make a really positive difference to your birth experience.

Did you know?

Belly dancing dates back over 6,000 years and was originally a birth dance, "la dance du ventre"; the movements simulate and represent those used during birth to help the baby descend and to keep the muscles strong.

A baby is an angel whose wings decrease as his legs increase
– Author unknown

For the many thousands of women who have used the techniques, it is becoming clear that Natal Hypnotherapy

reaches the parts that other antenatal courses cannot reach – Irena Popiolek

It is great that you are reading this book, and I am sure you will agree that it all makes sense in theory; however, if you truly want to have a better birth experience, then you need to commit yourself to preparing, practising and believing.

The Natal Hypnotherapy approach is based on five simple steps:

1. **Overcoming fear**
   The first and most important step is to acknowledge and face your fears. By bringing your fears up to the surface now, they will not be your lurking "tiger" in the shadows, ready to pounce once you are in the vulnerable state of giving birth. In addition, practising Natal Hypnotherapy will ensure that your mind is clear of fears and that the language you use to yourself is positive and beneficial.

2. **Learning ways to deal with pain**
   Learning deep relaxation, breathing, and natural pain-management skills will help you cope with the sensations from contractions during birth. Knowing how to stay completely relaxed will naturally lead to less discomfort and more-effective Contractions.

3. **Knowing you can do it!**
   Pregnancy isn't an illness or a medical condition. Women have given birth since time began and your body is perfectly designed to do it. By taking birth out of your intellectual mind and giving it back to your birthing mind and body, you will become more confident and trusting that you are able to go through this instinctive process.

4. **Preparing your birth partner**
   Yes, you'll be doing most of the work, but don't underestimate the support of others. The more informed your partner is, the more he or she can help and play an active part in the birth. Make sure your birth partner is fully prepared and knows how to work effectively with both you and the medical team. Learn together so that you are both informed and confident!

Every child begins the world again – Henry David Thoreau

5. Acquiring practical skills

You don't have to be a passive "patient" when you give birth. There are all sorts of practical steps you can take to increase your control, confidence and focus. There are so many practical tips and exercises which will help you physically, as well as emotionally, during birth.

Characteristics of a Natal Hypnotherapy mother

All women are different and all labours are different. However, there are some common characteristics of the birthing experiences of women who use Natal Hypnotherapy:

- They may appear very calm, confident, quiet and focused.

- They will breathe deeply, quietly and rhythmically through contractions.

- They may appear to be in a trance-like state or in "the zone".

- It is not uncommon for women using Natal Hypnotherapy to be sent home, as they appear not to be in established labour.

- They may not appear to be in "pain" – this can be quite misleading for birth professionals, as they may not be able to tell from the woman's external appearance whether she is in "established labour".

- Their birth partners may be more calm and confident than others and may be taking more of a leading role with the birth professionals in order to allow the mother to focus and remain undisturbed.

By following the exercises in this book, listening to the dowloads or attending a course, **the benefits to you, your baby and your partner will be priceless:**

- You will be able to tap into the subconscious part of your mind to deal with, and overcome, any fear and anxiety associated with giving birth.

- By reducing, if not eliminating, the fear associated with birth, you will reduce the tension in your body, which will lower pain sensations to a manageable level.

Did you know?

When a Mum relaxes, her unborn baby does too. When pregnant women Listened to soothing music, researchers found that the baby's breathing and heart rate slowed down.

Experience is determined by yourself – not the circumstances of your life
– Gita Bellin

- You will learn to enter deep relaxation at will.

- You will learn effective breathing techniques – a useful life skill!

- You will learn specific pain-management techniques, similar to those used by dentists to perform surgery without anaesthesia.

- Being more relaxed and breathing effectively during the birth, you can more effectively maintain your energy levels, your blood pressure and the level of oxygen to your muscles.

- Effective breathing increases oxygen to your baby and improves the removal of both toxins and lactic acid build-up.

- During your pregnancy, you will take time out to relax on a regular basis.

- You will spend time bonding with your baby during your pregnancy.

- By absorbing positive suggestions about the birthing process and your body's ability to give birth, you will increase your level of self-confidence and trust in your body's natural ability to give birth.

- You will be less likely to require medical intervention or additional pain relief.

A mum's experience

"My labour came on very suddenly – I had one painful contraction at home, and the next few were three to four minutes apart. We went straight to hospital. It was a 20-minute drive and I listened to the track in the car. I was extremely relaxed and focused; my husband thought my contractions had stopped, as I was so quiet!

I was 10 cm dilated on admission to the labour ward and wanted to push straight away. My baby girl was born less than two hours after the first contraction, which was amazing after a long and difficult first labour that had ended with an emergency Caesarean under general anaesthetic. Natal Hypnotherapy™ helped me a great deal and I would recommend it to everybody."

Sarah Hawker, UK

The more you depend on forces outside yourself, the more you are dominated by Them – Harold Sherman

- Your contractions are likely to be more effective and so your labour is likely to be more manageable.

- If you have had a positive birth experience, your postnatal recovery is likely to be far quicker and easier. In addition, research has shown a reduction in the likelihood of suffering postnatal depression and an increased ability to breastfeed.

Your **baby** will also draw on the benefits of you being a relaxed and calm mother:

- Research has shown that babies will pick up on the hormones released by the mother and will absorb them as a blueprint for life. Therefore, the more relaxed a mother is during her pregnancy, the more the baby will be influenced in this way.

- If a mother is able to birth calmly and instinctively, the baby will be receiving high levels of oxygen and low levels of stress hormones.

- Babies born in this way tend to stay calm, quiet and alert once they are born.

- As there are lower risks, babies tend to have higher APGAR scores.

- Mother and baby have spent time bonding and communicating in the womb, which then continues in a natural, easy way once the baby is born.

Benefits to the birth partner:

- Increased confidence in your ability to support your partner.

- Understanding what your partner needs in order for her to birth instinctively.

- Learning practical tools and techniques to help you both during the birth.

- Learning tools to help you to stay calm and relaxed.

- Understanding your choices.

- Gaining the confidence to work with the medical team in a positive way.

By using the techniques described in this book, listening to the tracks or attending one of the courses (see appendix for more details), you will gradually replace your old beliefs, fears and thoughts about birth with ones which are positive, empowering, instinctive and calm, so that you become both consciously and subconsciously convinced that you can trust your body to birth instinctively.

A baby is God's opinion that life should go on – Carl Sandburg

What is the evidence that it works?

Clinical research[1] has shown that for women using hypnosis for birth there is a:

Reduction in length of labour	Studies showed a reduction from 9.3 hours to 6.4 hours for first-time mums, and from 6.2 hours to 5.3 hours for second-time + mums
Less reported pain	Mothers gave an average of 6 on a self-scoring model of 0–10, with 10 being the highest
Reduction in medical intervention and use of forceps or ventouse	Studies reported an 84–99% rate of spontaneous, non-surgical deliveries
Reduced Caesarean rate	Studies reported Caesarean rates of between 5 and 8% compared with the national average of 24%
Reduced need for pharmacological anaesthesia/analgesia	Studies reported a 55–79% rate of non-medicated births
In addition, research showed that, for women who used hypnosis but then needed chemical anaesthetics, the anaesthetics were administered more easily, and smaller amounts were needed to have the same clinical effect.	

[1] **Sources**
1.   Jenkins, M. W., Pritchard M. H., Aberdare District Maternity Unit, Mid Glamorgan, Wales. *Br J Obstet Gynaecol*, 1993 Mar; 100(3): 221–6.
2.   Harmon T. M., Hynan M. T., Tyre T. E., The University of Wisconsin, Milwaukee, *J Consult Clin Psychol*, 1990 Oct; 58(5):525–30.
3.   Alice A. Martin, PhD; Paul G. Schauble, PhD; Surekha H. Rai, PhD; and R. Whit Curry, Jr, MD, Gainesville, Florida, *The Journal of Family Practice* • MAY 2001 • Vol. 50, No. 5 General.
4.   Schauble P. G., Werner W. E., Rai S. H., Martin A., Counseling Center, University of Florida, Gainesville, Florida. *American Journal of Clinical Hypnosis*, 1998 Apr; 40(4):273–83.
5.   August, R. V., Obstetric hypnoanesthesia. *American Journal of Obstetrics and Gynecology*, 79, 1131–1137, 1960, and August, R. V., *Hypnosis in Obstetrics*. New York: McGraw Hill, 1961.

Aim to do the thing you think you cannot do – Eleanor Roosevelt

A mum's experience

"Matthew is my second baby, my first being born by emergency C-section after five days of labour (failed induction). The C-section had gone wrong: I felt the incisions during the C-section, and then the wound was infected for six months and needed packing every day ... It was terrible. I was very keen not to repeat any of this bad experience the second time around.

I learnt Natal Hypnotherapy at home and found I was able to deal with and let go of my bad C-section experience. The techniques helped me to put all the negative feelings behind me, and I was able to start on a fresh birth plan for Matthew.

Matthew was one week overdue, so they decided to induce me again. After two pessaries, I went into labour, and 2 hours 40 minutes later Matthew was born. I used a TENS machine, gas and air, and Natal Hypnotherapy. I stood up for 80% of my labour, and as Matthew's heartbeat was not good I had ventouse for speed. Four pushes later and Matthew was born!

Throughout my labour I repeated all the time, '3, 2, 1, relax, Jane', which really helped me to slow down the pain.

I asked for a private space to labour in (my own baobab tree!) and was given a side room, so I had the lights off, the window open for fresh air and quiet, and the door closed. Just me and my husband. When I did go down to the delivery suite, I felt in control, and I was able to tell the midwife what I wanted. As Matthew became a bit distressed, they wanted to give me a C-section, but I trusted my body and asked for extra time. Very soon I started to push when I felt the urge (much to the surprise of the midwife).

I feel that Natal Hypnotherapy gave me back control and provided me with the tools to help me cope with whatever happened."

Jane Thompson, UK

Be miserable, or motivate yourself. Whatever has to be done, it's always your choice
– Wayne Dyer

Chapter 6 – Understanding hypnosis and how it can help

Before we go into more depth on Natal Hypnotherapy skills and techniques, it is useful to have a little background on hypnosis: what it is, what it is used for, and how it works. Many couples who learn and practise Natal Hypnotherapy realise that this is actually a skill for life that they can use in many other areas of their lives.

A dad's experience

"I came on a Natal Hypnotherapy course a couple of weeks ago with my wife. Even though I was a real sceptic about hypnosis (to be honest I was quite wary about it after seeing a show at college), we both loved the course and it put aside all my concerns.

However, the main reason for me writing to you is that I wanted to let you know that I learnt so much more than I had bargained for! We live in Luxembourg and we always drive to and from the UK due to my fear (well, former fear!) of flying.

After everything we learnt on the course I decided that it was not only Linda who could benefit, but that I could use the techniques to sort out some of my fears. So I decided to put it into practice for myself, and wrote myself a script to help with my fear of flying. I recorded the script and then listened to it every night for a week. Yesterday I flew for the first time in ages and, miraculously, I was fine.

I am so amazed and totally convinced that hypnotherapy can truly help make things happen."

Andrew Jackson, Luxembourg

To find yourself, think for yourself – Socrates

Hypnosis through time

Hypnosis has been used in different guises in almost all cultures. Over 4,000 years ago, the founder of Chinese medicine, Wang Tai, used words as healing tools, while druids used "magic sleep", and hieroglyphics on Egyptian tombs show sleep chambers as healing centres. Even Hippocrates, the father of medicine, said:

> The affliction suffered by the body, the soul sees quite well with the eyes shut.[1]

In the Bible there are references to techniques akin to the use of hypnosis, such as the power of the word, changing beliefs, overcoming fear and changing life long behaviours. In fact, it could be argued that many miracles that happened "within" people can be attributed to the use of hypnotic language to instil new beliefs and expectations:

> So the Lord caused a deep sleep to fall upon man and while he slept took one of his ribs and closed up this place with flesh.[2]

In this example, it could be argued that God used hypnosis as an anaesthetic so that Adam felt no pain during the removal of his rib. Another example is the many cases of healing taking place from the words spoken to the sufferer:

> This man was listening to Paul as he spoke, who when he had fixed his gaze upon him, and had seen that he had faith to be made well, said with a loud voice, 'Stand upright on your feet.' And he leaped up and began to walk.[3]

One of the most famous practitioners of hypnosis, and the first to try to understand how hypnosis worked, was Franz Anton Mesmer (hence the word mesmerism), who developed his theory and practice in the 1700s. He was mainly interested in using what he called "animal magnetism" to help cure people of ills. Even he recognised the benefit of this for women in childbirth when he suggested in 1784 that women should not need to suffer pain during childbirth. Mesmer was later discredited, as he used theatrical and dramatic displays to prove his theories.

However, others followed in his path as they began to realise that it was not the theatrics that brought about the healing in people, but the

Did you know?

The word hypnosis comes from the Greek word "hypnos" meaning to sleep. This is itself a misnomer, as, in hypnosis, you are not actually asleep. The term was originally "neuro hypnosis" or "sleep of the nervous system".

Thoughts are things – they have tremendous powers – Bryan Adams

trance-like state that people seemed to enter into. This state could easily be entered into by asking the subject to relax and empty their mind of thoughts. Once in this state, the subject was able to use the power of their mind to create different feelings and even experience tastes and smells.

By the mid-nineteenth century a recognised surgeon, Dr. James Braid, coined the phrase "neuro-hypnosis" or "sleep of the nervous system" (after the Greek god of sleep, Hypnos), as he noticed that people in hypnosis appeared to be asleep when in a trance-like state. He used hypnosis as a form of pain relief in his work between 1840 and 1850.

However, it was the work of Scotsman James Esdaile which is most impressive – he recorded using hypnosis as a form of anaesthesia in over 2,000 minor and 300 major operations, including 19 amputations and the removal of testicular cancer[4].

By 1892, the British Medical Association first recognised the use of hypnosis as a therapeutic agent. Unfortunately, with the introduction of chloroform, the popularity of hypnosis as an anaesthetic began to wane. However, around this time, the use of hypnosis took a different turn when it was used to help deal with emotional and psychological issues by leading figures such as Sigmund Freud, the founder of psychoanalysis.

Through his *Studies on Hysteria* (1895) Freud introduced a very different therapeutic use for hypnosis. Freud held the controversial belief that many physical and most mental problems in adult life are caused by unconsciously repressed memories and desires. He used hypnosis to help people re-experience their childhood memories (regression) in order to discharge associated negative emotions (catharsis) and thereby achieve experiential insight into their unconscious.

Freud's practices of direct suggestion and regression therapy are still the two main forms of hypnotherapy used today. Currently, hypnosis is used and applied in a wide variety of areas, from dealing with post-traumatic stress to overcoming phobias and curing obsessive-compulsive disorders.

The secret of making something work in our lives is first of all the deep desire to make it work, then the faith and belief that it can work – Eileen Caddy

The use of hypnosis in childbirth

Returning to the use of hypnosis for childbirth, hypnotherapy has been used more formally for over 100 years, and there are many examples of its use across the world.

In the 1920's in the former USSR, the hypnosis pioneer Platonov became well known for his hypno-obstetric successes. In fact, Stalin was so impressed by this approach that he later set up a nationwide programme headed by Velvoski, who combined hypnosis with Pavlovian techniques to help women manage childbirth[5]. These methods were then developed by Fernand Lamaze, who later created the Lamaze technique.

Obstetrician Dr. Joseph B. DeLee advocated in the 1930s that hypnosis was the "only anaesthetic without danger" and told his profession:

> I am irked when I see my colleagues neglect to avail themselves of this harmless and potent remedy.

In the UK, many doctors used hypnosis, not only for helping women with labour, but also whilst performing Caesarean sections. Hospitals across Russia in the 1950s routinely used hypnosis and psychoprophylaxis, which was seen as a low-cost and simple approach to reducing chemical pain relief[6].

Since the 1960s in the US, there has been an increase in interest in the use of hypnosis in obstetrics, with many doctors and hypnotherapists supporting, endorsing and practising the techniques.

These have been backed up by research, papers and books by Erickson (1967), Kroger (1970), a gynaecologist and obstetrician specialising in hypnosis for birth who wrote *Childbirth with Hypnosis* (and, incidentally, whose mother was attended by Joseph B. DeLee at his birth), Goldmann (1990), Bowers (1981), Cheek (1975), Barnett (1984), Davidson (1962), Mellegren (1966), Abramson & Heron (1950) and Werner (1970), who have done a great deal to increase the credibility of the use of hypnosis in childbirth.

Did you know?

Studies at Stanford University showed that intelligence or IQ had no bearing on the ability to practise hypnosis. This dispels the myth that you need to be weak minded or have a low IQ to be good at hypnosis.

We are what we think – all that we are arises with our thoughts –
The Dhammapada

For example, Werner delivered over 6,000 babies using chemical anaesthesia before discovering hypnosis, after which he went on to support over 3,000 women to give birth using hypnosis.

In fact, it was predominantly the work of Dr. Milton Erickson in the USA in the 1950s which changed the medical opinion of hypnotherapy and so helped to legitimise it, first in 1955, when the use of hypnosis as a form of pain relief was once again recognised and approved by the British Medical Association, which stated that:

> *Did you know?*
>
> Hypnotherapy was recognised as a valuable therapy by the British Medical Association (BMA), first in 1892 and then again in 1955.

> *Hypnosis is an effective method of relieving pain in birth without altering the normal course of labour.*

This was closely followed by the approval of the American Medical Association in 1958.

So, what exactly is hypnosis?

In spite of this long and credible history, for many people today, the term "hypnosis" conjures up all kinds of images, from swinging pendulums to people acting like chickens on stage. There are many misperceptions of what hypnosis is and what it is not. Ironically, even Grantly Dick-Read was wary of hypnosis and believed that it was taking away a woman's control.

However, as more and more research is done into the efficacy of hypnosis (many items of research can be found on PubMed, the world's largest database of medical research), there is growing acceptance and awareness of the connection with our thoughts and the way our bodies function. As a result, hypnosis is being recognised and is gaining credibility.

There is a great deal of myth and misunderstanding surrounding the word and the uses of hypnosis. If ever there was a word which has caused confusion and misunderstanding, it is this – even the Greek origin of the word, "hypnos", meaning to sleep, is inappropriate in this context. Most people's perceptions of hypnosis come from what they have seen on films and TV, from the Svengali and the pendulum-swinging circus act to Paul McKenna's stage shows.

First and foremost, hypnosis is a completely natural state of being – in fact, you have already experienced it thousands of times. It is a pleasant state of mental relaxation during which you are still aware of what is going on around you, but have mentally "gone

A man's character may be learned from the adjectives which he habitually uses in conversation – Mark Twain

somewhere else" or "are away with the fairies". The phrase "the lights are on, but no one's home" comes to mind.

It is a time when you are taking a step away from the here and now and drifting into a different "zone". The state is similar to daydreaming or to when you are doing something repetitive or therapeutic. It is a time when you are not thinking with your rational, analytical and critical mind, but instead your mind is "wandering or drifting".

For example, have you ever driven somewhere, only to realise that you cannot remember a single thing about the journey? You had "gone" somewhere in your mind, yet you were still able to drive safely.

Or have you been so engrossed in a book that you have lost track of time or have not heard when someone has called you?

In both of these examples, you were not asleep or under the control of someone else, but in a hypnotic state. You were still conscious and able to function, but your mind had drifted off to thoughts unconnected to the activity you were doing. That is to say that there was a degree of communication between the two different parts of your mind, which we will call the conscious and the subconscious.

The conscious is the higher-thinking, rational, analytical, decision-making part of you. The subconscious is the instinctive, emotive, animalistic part of you which stores everything that has ever happened to you.

Being in a hypnotic state diminishes the conscious, analytical, rational part of the mind in order to improve communication with the subconscious, emotional part of the mind. We naturally dip in and out of these two parts hundreds of times a day, so there is always communication between them. Mostly, however, we are not consciously "in control" of that communication.

As this type of hypnotic experience is a completely natural event, which everyone experiences, it is difficult to give an exact definition of it. However, here are a few key characteristics of natural hypnosis:

Did you know?

You have already experienced the state of hypnosis thousands of times!

It is that time when you are aware of your surroundings but your mind has "wandered off", as your thoughts are focused on something other than the action you are currently doing.

Love is giving someone your undivided attention – Author unknown

- It happens all the time that you are awake.
- You are usually not aware of this communication.
- The quality or depth of this natural hypnosis will vary considerably.
- Everyone experiences natural hypnotic states many times a day.

In summary, being in a hypnotic state is simply a time when you have some or all of the following:

1. You are deeply relaxed.
2. You are very focused on one thing.
3. Your mind "wanders".
4. You feel a bit distanced from your actual surroundings.
5. Time passes in an illogical way.
6. You become open to positive suggestions.

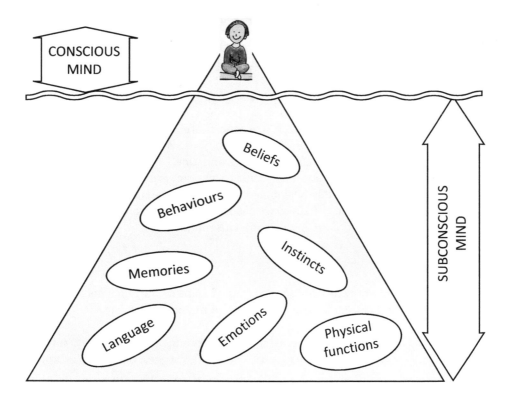

God sends children to enlarge our hearts, and make us unselfish and full of kindly sympathies and affections – Mary Howitt

So, as you can now see, everyone enters into the state of hypnosis many times a day. If nature had its way and we lived in a calm, non-pressurised society, we would naturally be in a hypnotic state for approximately twenty minutes every hour and a half (study by Ernest Rossi, American psychologist).

The benefits to this way of being are immeasurable – lower blood pressure, increased energy, a better-functioning body, calmer thoughts, better sleep, the ability to deal with situations more effectively, etc. In our modern society we hardly ever allow ourselves the time out to get into a hypnotic, relaxed state, and so often our bodies begin to suffer – a point in case is the drastically rising rate of stress-related illnesses.

These experiences are known as "natural hypnosis". What most people are unsure about or want to know more about is what is called "intended hypnosis". This is when you use the state of hypnosis for a specific outcome – you have a goal in mind, such as relaxation, pain relief, or overcoming a phobia, and you use the state of hypnosis to help you achieve it.

Intended hypnosis

Hypnosis, and the use of the state of hypnosis, allows us to actively communicate between the conscious and subconscious with a particular purpose in mind.

A definition by Alman and Lambrou states that:

> Hypnosis is a state of mind in which suggestions are acted upon much more powerfully than is possible under normal conditions. While in hypnosis, one suppresses the power of the conscious criticism. One's focus of attention is narrower and one's level of awareness on a focal point is much higher than if one were awake. During this heightened focus and awareness, suggestions appear to go directly into the subconscious … You can control areas yourself that are normally out of reach of your conscious mind.[7]

According to the Hypnotherapy Association:

> Using hypnosis, whereby the subconscious mind can be contacted, inner power can be harnessed to promote desired change and physical well being.[8]

Intended hypnosis is the active process of connecting into the part of the mind responsible for all change. In this state, your conscious mind is not blocking suggestions, so the subconscious

Babies touch the world with love – Author unknown

mind is totally receptive and is therefore much more likely to succeed in making the desired changes. This is far more effective than relying on determination and willpower, which is what most people rely upon to make changes.

Researchers and scientists who have studied hypnosis recognise that the state of hypnosis has special qualities. When you are in this state you can control areas of yourself that are normally out of reach of your conscious mind. This includes controlling bodily functions, such as slowing down your heart rate, stopping bleeding, controlling anxiety and reducing pain.

What is the difference between hypnosis, self-hypnosis and hypnotherapy?

It is useful to clarify this, as many people are still under the impression that hypnosis is something done to you when you are under someone else's control.

Essentially all hypnosis is self-hypnosis. A hypnotherapist may be able to guide you with the use of his words; however, each person is completely in control of their own mind and only you

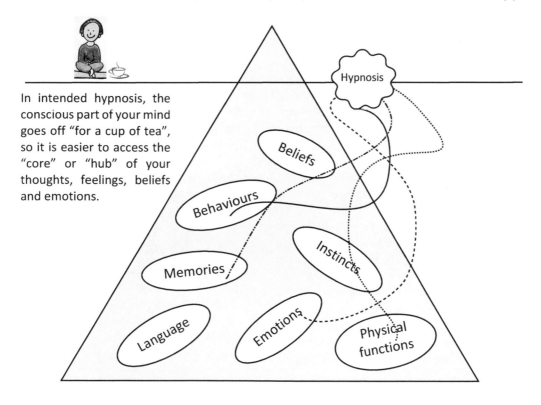

In intended hypnosis, the conscious part of your mind goes off "for a cup of tea", so it is easier to access the "core" or "hub" of your thoughts, feelings, beliefs and emotions.

All that I am or hope to be, I owe to my angel mother – Abraham Lincoln

can decide which suggestions and visualisations to follow. You are in complete control of where your mind takes you.

Even when a therapist or a MP3 is taking you through a visualisation, it is still up to you how you interpret that visualisation and whether you really want to follow what is being said. For example, you may hear a visualisation of a beach, but only you can decide which beach, what it looks like, who you are with, and so on. You may even choose not to go to a beach or find it difficult to visualise a beach, and may just feel colours or hear sounds. Again, you are in control.

In the same way, if there is something that you do not agree with, then your subconscious mind will not accept or take on board the suggestions.

The term hypnotherapy is made up of two words – hypnosis and therapy. Hypnosis itself is not a treatment – it is a state of being (as seen above). The state itself is very similar to meditation and is beneficial in that it is deeply relaxing, helps you focus, and encourages you to take quiet time and simply to "be".

Hypnotherapy is the use of hypnosis for a therapeutic end. It involves using the intended state of hypnosis and applying therapeutic suggestions, metaphors and other techniques to bring about a positive change.

With hypnotherapy you are communicating with the part of the mind responsible for all change. As you are dealing directly with the subconscious, you are able to influence and convince the part of you responsible for behaviour, beliefs, language, etc that there is a better or new way of doing things, and this then becomes your new reality or new way of doing something.

As a result, using hypnosis to bring about changes can be so much more effective than relying on determination and willpower, which are in the domain of the conscious.

It is often old memories, fears, beliefs and patterns of behaviour which dictate how we respond to the world today, no matter how out of date or inappropriate they may be. In a way, hypnotherapy is a way to "update" the subconscious so that it is working more effectively and with a more positive outcome than before. As the subconscious part of our mind is where we store our fears and patterns of behaviour, by tapping

Did you know?

There are over 11,000 research studies on hypnosis and hypnotherapy cited on PubMed – the world's largest database on scientific research.

Parents who are afraid to put their foot down usually have children who tread on their toes – Chinese proverb

into that part of the mind we can change or overcome these elements to help us deal more effectively with the world around us (see next chapter for more on how the mind works).

What can hypnotherapy be used for?

The range of things which hypnotherapy has been successfully used for is absolutely vast, and yet, in clinical and medical terms, we have only scratched the surface.

Hypnotherapy has been scientifically proven as a treatment for a great many medical and psychological conditions. Artists and poets, such as André Breton and the early Surrealists, have used it for inspiration and self-exploration.

Performers like Sylvester Stallone, Daryl Hannah, Gareth Gates and Orlando Bloom use hypnosis to improve their performance and to develop their creativity. A great many top athletes and sports professionals, such as Tiger Woods, now improve their sporting performance using hypnosis.

Salesmen, trainers and managers often use it to increase their business success. Mystical, spiritual, and religious people of every creed and culture, from ancient times to the present day, have used the techniques of hypnosis alongside their traditional prayer and meditation.

In the field of medicine and pain management, hypnosis has been proven to help with hundreds of different issues, from reducing hot flushes in breast-cancer survivors to pain management and managing asthma.

There are thousands of other research studies which have shown that this Kindofvisualisationandpositivesuggestion leads to high success rates in almost all fields of activity, from academic performance to mountain climbing and athletics.

A well-known study on creative visualisation in sports involved Russian scientists and coaches.

Did you know?

Famous people who have used hypnosis to help them overcome fears, phobias and behavioural challenges include:

- Orlando Bloom to stop a chocolate craving
- Kevin Costner to overcome seasickness
- Tiger Woods to help improve his golf
- Nicole Ritchie for the birth of her first child

Never try to make your son or daughter another you – one is enough!
– Arnold Glasow

Prior to the 1980 Olympics, they compared four groups of Olympic athletes in terms of their training schedules:

- Group 1 – 100% physical training
- Group 2 – 75% physical training with 25% mental training
- Group 3 – 50% physical training with 50% mental training
- Group 4 – 25% physical training with 75% mental training

Group 4, with 75% of their time devoted to mental training, performed the best. Group performance level fell right in order – as mental training increased, performance increased. The Soviets discovered that mental images can act as a prelude to muscular impulses.

Hypnosis has been used by countless thousands of people to help them in dealing with the everyday problems of living: to overcome fears and inhibitions, to develop skills, and to cultivate self-esteem and confidence. Most of all, hypnosis liberates the natural potential of the mind for self-actualisation and personal empowerment!

In summary:

Hypnosis is a pleasant state of mental relaxation.

- It is **not** like being asleep or unconscious.
- It is a natural state with no negative side effects.
- You are under your own control, **not** anyone else's.
- Hypnosis is well recognised in medicine and psychology.
- Everyone can learn to enter hypnosis or self-hypnosis.

Characteristics of natural hypnosis:

- Natural hypnosis is the communication between two levels of your mind.
- It happens all the time that you are awake.
- You are usually not aware of this communication.
- The quality of this natural hypnosis will vary considerably.
- Everyone experiences natural hypnotic states many times a day.
- The best communication and hypnosis is when we are relaxed and the conscious mind is less active – daydreaming, for example.
- There is also powerful communication between the two levels when we experience intense emotion.

Parents learn a lot from their children about coping with life – Muriel Spark

Intended hypnosis is:

- Using natural hypnosis with awareness.
- Gives you a guaranteed depth.
- Is a safe way to access your subconsious.
- Is focused relaxation.
- The use of your mind and imagination to create a desired change within yourself.

---

[1] Temes, Roberta, 2000, *The Complete Idiot's Guide to Hypnosis*, Alpha Books, p. 54.

[2] Janet Fricker & John Butler, 2001, *Secrets of Hypnotherapy*, Dorling Kindersley, 2001.

[3] *The Bible*, Acts 14: 9–10.

[4] Milne Bramwell, J., 1909, *Hypnotism and Treatment by Suggestion*, London, Cassell.

[5] Gérard V. Sunnen, M.D., 1999, *Miscellaneous Medical Applications of Hypnosis*, Bellevue Hospital and New York University.

[6] Paula Michaels, "On The Trail of Dr. Lamaze: A Transnational History of Childbirth Education, 1930–80", http://www.irex.org/programs/stg/research/05/michaels.pdf.

[7] Alman, B. & Lambrou, P., 1983, *Self Hypnosis – The Complete Manual for Health and Self Change*.

[8] www.thehypnotherapyassociation.co.uk

Each day of our lives we make deposits in the memory banks of our children
– Charles R. Swindoll

mum's experience

"I had originally planned to use a birth centre, but Natal Hypnotherapy made me feel so relaxed and in control before the birth that we decided on a home birth.

My waters went at 6.50 p.m. and contractions started about 7.30 p.m. Things progressed at an amazing rate, with contractions coming every four to five minutes by about 10 p.m. I called the midwife, who suggested that we wait another hour; we later found out that she thought I was too calm for things to be so far progressed. I definitely think midwives should ask if mums are using hypnotherapy. I got in the bath, which helped, but got out and called the midwife again, as the contractions were now coming every three to four minutes and were really intense. I knew things were happening, so insisted they send the midwife.

All this time I was using a combination of golden-light relaxation breathing and visualisation. At this point I was visualising my contractions as waves. When they got more intense, I visualised myself climbing a mountain. I also took myself to my special place quite frequently. The midwife arrived around 12 a.m., expecting to check me and go home, as I was still very calm. She went a shade of white when she examined me to find I was 6–7 cm dilated, as she hadn't brought the gas and air or much of the necessary equipment with her!

She made a phone call immediately for the second midwife, who did not arrive until 2 a.m., as she had to come from far away. I was well into transition by the time the second midwife arrived. Again, the hypnotherapy really helped, and I was able to visualise my baby sliding down the birth canal. All in all, the whole birth experience was amazing. The combination of many weeks of yoga and many listens to the hypnotherapy track meant that I was calm and prepared and that my subconscious knew what was going on, even though it was my first time.

As a result, I didn't panic, and that's why I think things went so smoothly and quickly. The pain never really got too much and actually I did find myself occasionally finding it pleasurable, as the track suggested I might. At many times during the labour I heard the MP3 voice in my head, which encouraged me to think that everything was as it should be."

Sarah Pryor, UK

Chapter 7 – How the mind works

Creating our subconscious

Think of your mind as being a bit like a computer.

From the time babies begin growing in the womb, all their experiences are being logged in the database in their own 'personal computer', known as their mind or subconscious. All through the baby and childhood years, their main preoccupation is to have their basic needs met and so ultimately to survive. As all their experiences are being stored and monitored, any experiences which equate to danger or not having their needs met are effectively noted and marked in red. These situations are stored in a special file and are highlighted to ensure that they avoid the same situation happening or at least have a coping mechanism to deal with it more effectively in the future.

A child learns what is socially acceptable, what is right and wrong (in her family culture) and which actions trigger a negative or a positive response. Basically she is creating an immensely complex computer program which she will use and refer to for the rest of her life. The sum of her experiences dictate her way of behaving, her way of thinking, her triggered responses, her fears and aspirations.

The mind is particularly good at recalling experiences and responses to negative situations. Because the mind wishes to protect us at all times from feeling pain, fear, humiliation, rejection, and so on, the responses learnt to protect us as children may stay with us through-out our lives, long after the actual circumstances or situations have changed.

For example, if a child was bullied at school, he may become reclusive, shy, wary of people. To help protect himself, these characteristics

Did you know?

All our memories and behaviours are stored not just in the brain but in cells around our body. People who have had organ transplants have found that they have taken on new memories, new likes and dis-likes, and even new behaviours and ways of thinking!

A baby is born with a need to be loved – and never outgrows it!
– Frank A. Clark

may stay with him long after he has left school and is no longer in a situation where he may be bullied.

Many painful emotions are caused by experiences and attitudes which were formed a long time ago, and so are in essence out of date and inappropriate for your life today. Many people often lose sight of the fact, or do not realise, that these reactions are being governed by out-of-date emotions and not by the situation in the here and now, as if they have not "upgraded the software".

Of course, many of these childhood protection mechanisms can change as you become an adult. However, for those that do not, hypnosis can be an incredibly useful tool to help "go in" and update the responses and rationale behind certain behaviours. Just like on your computer, you can upgrade the software, delete obsolete files, resort the filing system and archive old files. Using hypnosis, you can upgrade your system to make it more current, efficient and applicable to your life's situations in the here and now.

Opening the door to your mind

So how can you get access to all those old files?

Using a different analogy, you may like to imagine that your mind is like the floor plan of a house. The conscious part of your mind is the front entrance hall or porch, which has a door leading to the rest of the house. Imagine that there is a doorman or security guard at the front entrance hall who is responsible for letting in, or keeping out, everything you experience. He or she is the gatekeeper, the protector, and most of the time the door to the house is guarded.

Behind the closed door is the rest of the house, which is like the subconscious – the huge part which stores all your memories, beliefs, patterns of behaviour, physical responses, etc.

Normally, the door is closed and the guard is on duty to protect you and to evaluate what you allow in and out of the house.

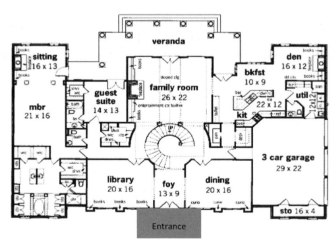

Education commences at the mother's knee, and every word spoken within the hearing of little children tends towards the formation of character – Hosea Ballou

However, when you daydream or are in a hypnotic state, the guard goes off for a tea break or a nap and the door opens, so you have access to wander freely around the rest of the house. As your mind stores all your memories, thoughts and feelings, the house can be huge!

Hypnosis can be particularly helpful, as it enables you to consciously send your guard on a tea break. You can then open the door to your subconscious and have a wander around your house without your guard looking over your shoulder analysing, criticising or rationalising. This gives you access to lots of rooms (memories, beliefs, emotions, etc) where you are then able to help re-educate, re frame or turn off responses which are no longer relevant, useful or in perspective.

Some rooms are bright and sunny and store positive memories. Others may be small, dark, under the cupboard or in the attic, and store negative memories and beliefs. Throughout our life the door is also thrown open when intense emotions are present such as fear, sadness or guilt. These experiences are then stored and a message is given to the guard to find a way to protect you from experiencing those feelings again.

As a result, the guard creates a coping strategy which he attaches to the experience as a way to help keep you safe. That experience is then locked away in a room which remains closed until a similar experience happens again, which triggers off the coping strategy or the response mechanism. At that point the trigger is so strong that it can override the conscious, rational response, which becomes powerless.

Sometimes, the subconscious will create an overprotective coping mechanism to avoid being put in that situation again – this can be the start of fears or more extreme phobias. An example would be a person involved in a car crash after driving for twenty years – the emotions of fear, pain and helplessness may trigger off a defence mechanism which says "being in a car is dangerous". Later, this trigger may get so strong that the person no longer feels safe and so refuses to get in a car, in spite of their conscious mind saying, "Don't be so silly – it was a fluke; it was an accident, and you have driven every day for twenty years and never had a problem."

Generally, any problems we have involve emotions that are inappropriate and excessive for the situation concerned, whether they be issues about confidence, weight, habits, presentation techniques or fear of childbirth. Using positive suggestions in hypnosis, you can "talk" directly to the part of you that is responsible for dealing with a particular situation and give it a new set of more realistic guidelines, a new coping strategy.

Children are a poor man's wealth – Danish proverb

This could include creating new patterns and altering the perspective of possibility and probability – i.e., it is possible that bad things can happen, but it is highly probable that they will not. Millions of people drive every day – the probability of having an accident is very, very small. If this is said at a conscious level, it will not be accepted, but at a subconscious level it is far more likely to be accepted.

Creating new patterns

Throughout life we are not stuck with all the same patterns: we are creating new patterns and new responses all the time. As well as good and useful responses, we often create new negative reactions to events as we go through life. Due to a particular set of circumstances, we can set up our own negative suggestions and triggers which bring about an undesirable effect.

An example is a father who comes home from work to his young family. Every time he sees the garage door go up (trigger) he begins to feel anxious. He knows he has to talk about some financial problems with his wife, that his two-year-old will be demanding attention, and that things need to be done around the house. As soon as he gets out of the car (trigger) he feels irritable and nervous and starts thinking of ways to avoid dealing with the family. As a result, the evenings are tense, fraught and stressful.

Using hypnosis he is able to change the negative triggers into positive ones. He is able to give a new set of instructions to his subconscious: for example, driving home is "his time" and allows him to think about and digest the day's activities; seeing the house (trigger) reminds him of how lucky he is to have such a wonderful family; opening the garage door (trigger) encourages him to think of each evening as a new opportunity to make the most of family life; getting out of the car (trigger) represents stepping out of his work mode and into his home mode, etc. After a few days he feels much more relaxed, is able to discuss his issues with his wife, and still finds time to play with his son.

What had changed? Only his perception and attitude.

Did you know?

When your baby is born, their brain will weigh about 350–400 grams and will have almost all the brain cells they will ever have. In fact, their brain will be closer to its full adult size than any other organ in their body.

Motherhood has a very humanising effect. Everything gets reduced to essentials –
Meryl Streep

Altering perspectives

In all of life's situations there are two elements – one is the actual situation and the second is our perspective of, or attitude towards, it. As a child, many of the perceptions, attitudes and beliefs you have will have been directed by those of your parents. However, beliefs are not rigid and cast in stone. As you become an adult, you can choose to hold onto your parents' perceptions of the world or to take responsibility yourself and make your own choices as to how you will interpret and respond to each situation.

In life there are a great many situations when we cannot alter the reality, but we always have a choice as to how we deal with it. An example is two people who were paralysed in a car crash. The first felt angry and bitter and spent many years feeling resentful at becoming a cripple and having to spend the rest of his life in a wheelchair. The second felt sad for a while, then decided he would do the best he could with his new life and focused all his energy on becoming a Paralympic athlete, going on to take part in games all around the world.

Again, through the use of hypnosis, which bypasses the critical, conscious part of the mind, our attitude and perspective of the world can be altered and reframed to help us make more positive and beneficial choices and responses to the way we deal with life today.

The power of words

In hypnotherapy the most powerful tool that is used is the spoken word. The words we use, both to ourselves and others, are more powerful than most people imagine.

"Words are, of course, the most powerful drug used by mankind" – Rudyard Kipling

Remember we discussed the fact that we were essentially mammals, especially when it comes to birthing? Well, there are of course a few differences between us and our mammal cousins.

The biggest difference is our ability to communicate – to use words for ourselves and with those around us. Out of words come thoughts; out of thoughts come ideas; out of ideas come inventions; out of inventions comes "civilisation". The words we use and how we use them

Did you know?

Your brain is incapable of knowing the difference between something you have experienced for real and something that you have imagined. Your physiological responses to both will be the same.

I miss thee, my Mother! Thy image is still the deepest impressed on my heart
– Eliza Cook

drive our daily lives. How we think and how we speak to ourselves drives our behaviour. The words and ideas we hear from others create our belief systems.

Words are the foundation for the way we live our lives. By focusing in on the words you use to yourself, you can change your entire perspective of the world: you can help heal your body, you can change your belief patterns, and you can change how you see yourself in the world.

Simply changing words can change lives.

Words spoken by a great leader can be uplifting and empowering; they can cause people to act in remarkable ways – for good and for bad. For example, the speeches of Hitler created a completely new mindset, a new way of thinking, a new belief system that led to some of the greatest atrocities known to man. The words of Winston Churchill inspired and motivated a nation.

The carefully chosen words of a doctor to an ill patient can create a belief that the patient may then follow to the letter – again for good and bad. How you were spoken to by your parents, your teachers, and your school friends can influence how you act and feel about yourself for the rest of your life.

Words we hear around us have enormous influence on our decisions and patterns of behaviour. If someone were to shout "bomb" in a room – imagine the response! We turn the interpretation of words into energy – fear, pride, happiness, anger, joy, etc. If someone criticises you unfairly, you turn that negative feeling into energy; if someone tells you that you have done a great job, you turn that energy into a positive feeling. It is easier to understand this with words spoken to you, but most people underestimate the impact that the words they speak to themselves have on their own energy levels and energy resources.

The subconscious takes words very literally and can hold onto them for a life-

Did you know?

"Try" is a negative and useless word as it implies a great deal of effort but not a lot of success – it is an excuse for failure, as you can claim to have "tried your best".

Think of these phrases:
"trying to conceive"
"trying to lose weight"
"I will try and breastfeed"

These would work far better by saying:
"I am preparing to conceive"
"I am starting to reduce my weight"
"I intend on breastfeeding"

What is done to children, they will do to society – Karl Menninger

time, especially words spoken by an authority figure in a frightening or intimidating way – "you are a greedy child – you will always be fat" "mark my words you will come to nothing", "pull yourself together – boys don't cry", "all the women in our family have terrible births".

These off-the-cuff comments can literally be im-printed into the mind of a child and stay with them through their adult years, affecting their ability to lose weight, to be a success, to show emotions, give birth, and so on.

Did you know?

The brain continues to produce new neurons throughout our lives, and it does so in response to thought and behaviour stimulation. Therefore, we can continue to learn new ways of doing things, new facts, new behaviours, and so on, throughout our lives.

Quite often, the words we speak to ourselves are based on these out-of-date or untrue assumptions, usually "ingrained" in us over time by parents, family culture, teachers, etc. If you are told enough times that you are stupid, careless, clumsy, worthless, then, sure enough, that is what you feel and that is how you speak to yourself. On the other hand, if you are told, or tell yourself, that you can do anything you set your mind to, you soon believe it. If the monologue in your mind is critical, judgmental, negative or blaming, the resulting feeling is one of guilt, anxiety, shame or fear. If the words are caring, loving, supportive and praising, the resulting feelings are those of confidence, self-esteem and positivity.

A positive attitude can have an immense impact on your physical, emotional and mental well-being. It can reduce stress and physical stress-related symptoms, including headaches, high blood pressure and digestive problems.

Based on the above, it is obvious that the words we hear at both the conscious and the subconscious level can influence how we deal with life around us. So, if we understand how much words can influence us in a negative way, think how the use of positive, uplifting, encouraging language can influence us in a positive way.

And this is even more the case when used with hypnosis. Because you are communicating directly with the subconscious, so much "harm" from words in the past can be undone and new ways of thinking can be installed.

Once you bring life into this world, you must protect it. We must protect it by changing the world – Elie Wiesel

What can I do to make sure hypnosis works for me?

Hypnosis can help install new programs, new videos, and new response mechanisms so that you can change the words you use to yourself and those around you with the intention of having a more successful, beneficial and useful outcome.

However, to really make changes, many factors are involved.

1. Motivation – the person really needs to want to change. Quite often there are reasons why we continue with the way we have done things even if they are not good for us, e.g. habits, patterns. These reasons are known as the "secondary gain" – it might be that you gain attention, sympathy, social acceptance, and so on. It is therefore important to understand what your secondary gain may be so that you can address that issue and find an alternative source.

2. A willingness to change – we are often stuck in patterns of behaviour because they keep us in our comfort zone. Change can take you out of that zone, which can be a bit scary for some. However, once the change has been made, you can often feel liberated and lighter knowing that you have made a positive choice to move forward in your life.

3. Trust in the therapist/approach – make sure that the person or approach you are working with is reputable and has a strong track record and good results. If you are working with an individual therapist, meet them before the session to make sure you feel at ease and comfortable with them. If not, then do not go ahead.

4. Time and commitment to practise hypnosis – as with any skill, the more you practise, the better the results you get. Occasionally, you can achieve great change with just one session, but usually it takes commitment and time to make the changes you want.

mum's experience

"I am sure that my positive pregnancy and birth experience would not have been possible without the Natal Hypnotherapy techniques taking away the "fear" of labour and pain. I never set out to have a natural labour and was convinced I would

Kids really brighten a household – they never turn off the lights – Ralph Bus

need pethidine at the very least. I also thought I would be the least-susceptible person to hypnosis, as I'm so manic; I never imagined I would be able to entirely manage my pain and the whole labour by concentrating on breathing, relaxing as much as possible, and reminding myself that this was nothing to be afraid of and that my body would manage this by itself.

I used the early Natal Hypnotherapy tracks to help me deal with a devastating miscarriage and then a fearful early pregnancy. Thankfully, everything went well and I began listening to the birth preparation one from about thirty-three weeks onwards. It helped me relax, but I never really believed it would be able to take away or help me control the pain of serious labour, as I'm a real wimp. I hoped, however, that it would get me through the initial stages so that when I got to hospital I could get some "proper" pain relief.

When my labour started I remained calm and relaxed, and focused on breathing; I relaxed as much as possible during and between contractions, and the suggestions from the track just came to me – that this was a natural, physical process and the feelings were just pressure, warmth and power, and nothing to be afraid of; that I should just leave it to my body and not worry about it. I thought I would stay at home as long as I felt able to manage the contractions, but, as I've said, I always intended to go into hospital for drugs when they became necessary.

I listened to the track constantly for about four hours, lying down in a dark room with my husband, using the '3, 2, 1, relax' technique – then, suddenly, I decided it was time to go to hospital. I don't know what changed, as the contractions were always bearable if I breathed through them, exhaled for as long as possible and relaxed, but I just wanted to go in.

When I got there I was amazed to be told that the baby's head was right there and I was ready to push! The midwives were amazed at how calm and relaxed I was, given this was a first baby, and that I'd managed the contractions and then the pushing without any drugs – I was even fully dressed at this point, having not had time to take off my shoes or jewellery! About ten minutes later my son was born, looking very lively and after a remarkably quick and painless labour. Thank you!"

Lindsay Whitehead, UK

Lucky parents who have fine children usually have lucky children who have fine parents – James A. Brewer

Chapter 8 – What is involved in a hypnotherapy session?

"An anxious mind cannot exist in a relaxed body"

Edmund Jacobson

For anyone experiencing hypnotherapy for the first time, there are bound to be some reservations and concerns. I would therefore like to take you, step by step, through the things that are likely to take place in a hypnosis session.

As stated before, anyone can enter into hypnosis and it is beneficial for everyone. However, it is important to feel confident in your therapist/approach, to want it to work and not to expect too much. For many people, they do not feel like they are in hypnosis and may even feel a little disappointed after the first session, as they may have heard every word, felt very aware of their surroundings and not "drifted off". All of that is OK and normal.

Whether you choose to go to see an individual therapist, go on a course, write your own script or use a CD, the process is likely to be very similar. The following steps will take place:

1. Setting the scene.
2. Induction.
3. Breathing and physical relaxation.
4. Deepener – guided imagery and visualisation.
5. Creating a special place.
6. Hypnotic suggestions.
7. Exit.

Peace does not mean to be in a place where there is no noise, trouble, or hard work. Peace means to be in the midst of all those things and still be calm in your heart – Marel Morin

1. Setting the scene

Before you begin, it is important that you:

- Have turned off all distractions, e.g. the phone.
- Are warm and comfortable.
- Understand that there is no right or wrong – there is nothing you have to do. It is simply a time to relax and enjoy the experience.
- Realise that hypnosis is not about achieving an empty mind – it is quite normal for thoughts to drift in and out. If you have thoughts, accept them and then let them drift away, while you return your attention to the sound of the therapist's voice.
- If you feel the need to move, scratch, sneeze, etc, then that is OK. It is not a game of musical statues!

2. Induction

This is the process which gently guides you away from your active conscious state and into a relaxed hypnotic state. It helps you slowly and steadily change your focus from the here-and-now reality, and into a more internal, focused and calm state. There are many ways to do this, which may include:

- Focusing all your attention on your breathing.
- Becoming aware of the feeling of different parts of your body.
- Counting backwards from 10 to 1.
- Imagining your mind has many levels – the highest is fully alert and awake, and the lowest is deep sleep; you imagine yourself going down one level at a time.

3. Relaxation and breathing

A key element to any hypnosis session is helping you to relax and breathe effectively. These are of course two of the most important and powerful techniques that you will learn when preparing for childbirth.

Did you know?

Deep breathing has been shown to reduce stress levels, reduce blood pressure, improve asthma, relieve pain, increase your body's immune system, increase flow of oxygenated blood and even help with weight loss.

A closed mind is like a closed book; just a block of wood – Chinese proverb

Everyone instinctively knows how to breathe. However, many people are not actually very good at making the most of each breath, nor do they know how to really use their breathing for their full benefit.

There are many different ways in which we breathe depending on our situation, exertion levels, stress levels, etc.

Normally, people's breathing is fairly shallow and rapid, involving only the chest expanding and contracting; however, the capacity of the ribs and chest to expand is quite limited.

Breathing deep down to your abdomen or diaphragm ensures that you get the maximum exchange of oxygen and release of carbon dioxide.

According to the renowned cardiologist Dr. Herbert Benson[1], slow, deep, rhythmic breathing triggers a physical relaxation response – the opposite to the "fight or flight" response. This relaxation response triggers a chain reaction of physical changes in your body. A slower heart rate increases blood flow to the extremities, muscular relaxation and increased absorption of oxygen. These things in themselves will increase a person's health and well-being, and of course will be especially beneficial during childbirth.

A deep, satisfying inhalation of breath activates the mind and body – oxygen stimulates the brain and feeds the cells throughout the body. Exhaling is a letting go – tension is released, carbon dioxide is expelled, and the muscles tend to relax even more during this part of the cycle.

4. Deepener – Guided imagery and visualisation

"The soul never thinks without a picture"
– Aristotle

The concept of depth of trance is the subject of considerable debate. Many people achieve wonderful results without ever feeling that "total blankness" that some relate to. One thing to really stress is that every person experiences hypnosis in a different way and that, again, there is no right or wrong. People can achieve incredible results from simply a few chosen words by a therapist without ever going into a deep trance-like state.

Did you know?

The use of visualisation, metaphor and storytelling has been around ever since humans were able to speak. Before books and writing, all learning was done through storytelling and metaphor.

A torn jacket is soon mended; but hard words bruise the heart of a child –
Henry Wadsworth Longfellow

However, for most people, there is a wonderful sense of relaxation and deepening during a hypnosis session. Many people do experience a feeling of sinking or going down, hence the use of the word "deep".

As a result, many people find the use of depth and the movement downwards a useful metaphor for reaching that state. This could be by imagining being in a lift and going down one floor at a time; or you could imagine that you are an autumn leaf or a feather floating down and down, or are walking down a staircase, etc.

Guided imagery is a wonderful way of encouraging your mind to step away from "reality" and into your own world of imagination. It increases your sense of focus and heightened awareness and helps you connect with the inner part of yourself.

A mum's experience

"My waters broke at 5.30 a.m., so we went into hospital to be checked. They sent us home as all was OK; however, by the time we got home, my contractions were very strong. As the midwives had advised that labour could go on for hours, I focused on making myself comfortable and prepared for a long day. By around midday I was labouring very hard; however, I thought I could not be in full labour, so I used my TENS machine on low and practised the relaxation and visualisation techniques learnt through the Natal tracks. Just before 3 p.m. I felt that I needed to go to hospital, but as I started to make my way to the car I stood up and felt the urge to push. We then discovered that my son's head was crowning. At 3 p.m. my son was born on our bedroom floor, with the paramedics arriving as his head was crowning.

I always felt that my pain threshold was very low; however, the tools really helped me manage the pain of labour. Having an unplanned home birth could have been very stressful and scary when I was in the latter stages of labour, but by taking myself away and visualising a safe place (as I had done listening to the track), I managed to have a very healthy and quick birth that I feel very positive about. I don't think I would have been so mentally prepared without these tools; they made me feel in control both physically and mentally in a really positive way. Thank you."

It is not because things are difficult that we do not dare; it is because we do not dare that they are difficult – Seneca

With guided imagery, it is important to remember that people all interpret the world in unique ways, and not everyone finds it easy to "visualise" or "see" things in their mind. Some people feel more comfortable "hearing" or "feeling" things, so a good therapist, and the most successful guided imagery, incorporates all the senses.

Another excellent tool in hypnosis is the use of metaphor, or figure of speech, concisely comparing two things. The mind can easily relate to and understand comparisons to stories, symbols or metaphors, even when the reality of the words may seem unconnected.

Some excellent examples are the "like/as if" group:

> *"feeling all stress melting away like butter melting in the sun; you are so limp and loose, as if you are a strand of overcooked spaghetti; all your muscles feel as if they have turned to jelly; feel yourself unwinding like the spring in a clock; let all your thoughts drift on by as if they are clouds in the sky."*

This kind of imagery is often used in hypnosis sessions.

5. Creating your special place

A technique often used in hypnosis is to encourage you to go to a "special place" in your mind. This is like having your own personal inner refuge, based on a real or imaginary place that you associate with relaxation, comfort, security, and peace. Maybe a room in your home, a cabin in the mountains ... a corner of your garden ... the warm sand of the beach, where you can hear the ocean waves coming to shore ... an open meadow full of wildflowers ... a soft, moss-carpeted spot in a peaceful woodland grove near a gentle brook.

By going to this place routinely when in hypnosis, it becomes easy and familiar to go to that place when you feel the need to relax and "get away" for a while. Many women who have practised this during their pregnancy find it a great tool to use during the birth. Even if the special place changes, the process is familiar.

> *Pretty much all the honest truth-telling there is in the world is done by children*
> *– Oliver Wendell Holmes*

A mum's experience

"I was totally zoned out – my whole focus had become internal as with every contraction I repeated '3, 2, 1, relax, Karen' to myself and in-between each contraction I went to my 'safe place', a beach I had been to on honeymoon in Malaysia. I remember scoffing at the point in the track where you describe the birth as being no more difficult than doing strenuous exercise, but that is exactly what it was like for me. It reminded me of doing the hill profile on the exercise bike where I just get my head down, turn my focus inwards and concentrate on breathing for the duration of the hill, then relax in the recovery stage.

I totally believe that the Natal Hypnotherapy kept me going a long way without pain relief and contributed greatly to the positive experience."

Karen Keast, N. Ireland

6. Hypnotic suggestions

This is where the real magic of hypnosis comes in, and what makes it different from meditation or general relaxation.

Once you are in a deeply relaxed state, you become far more open to positive suggestions. As we have already discovered, in a state of hypnosis, the power of the critical, analytical, conscious mind is greatly diminished, and the subconscious is more focused and more positive and thus more likely to accept suggestions made during this time.

Positive and post-hypnotic suggestions

The real magic behind hypnosis is the ability of the subconscious mind to listen to words and to translate them into new ways of thinking and responding.

Everything we do, every action we take in life, is triggered by something. Cause and effect. You are thirsty so you have a drink; your phone rings so you answer it; you feel angry so you shout; you feel stressed so you eat. And so on.

If you bungle raising your children, I don't think whatever else you do well matters very much – Jacqueline Kennedy Onassis

Did you know?

During labour, many women instinctively use their imagination to "go to" a safe place in their mind. The place may stay the same or it may change throughout the birthing. Your mind becomes very creative and you may be surprised at the images that your mind creates.

In the same way, so much of our unwanted behaviour is down to triggered responses based on our past experiences, e.g. eating because you are feeling a bit low, biting your nails because you are a bit bored, having a cigarette because you are a bit stressed. All those actions came from a cause. At a conscious level, we may not even be sure what the cause is and in many cases we find it very difficult, if not impossible, to change our reactions – which is why many habits are so difficult to give up.

However, when using hypnosis, you can help to retrain or re-programme your mind to provide a different and better response to the trigger – a new cause-and-effect situation.

This is done through the use of hypnotic and post-hypnotic suggestions. Direct hypnotic suggestions are related to things that you will do during the hypnosis session, such as close your eyes, become aware of your hands, imagine you are on a beach, relax your muscles, and so on. These are particularly useful if you are using hypnosis whilst going through a procedure such as dental work, having an injection, dealing with pain, etc.

However, if you are using hypnosis for stress management or birth preparation, then whilst you are in a hypnosis session, you are definitely relaxed, calm, breathing well and at ease. However, that does not reflect the "normal" situation that you know you will face in the future, such as being at work, on the tube, being in front of an audience or giving birth!

So it is the second type of suggestion, the post-hypnotic suggestion, where the real magic takes place, as this creates the change and effect you want for a time in the future.

A post-hypnotic suggestion is a suggestion given to an individual whilst they are in hypnosis, for an action or response to take place in the future, after the hypnotic experience has ended.

Like everything in life, a post-hypnotic suggestion is set up with a cause or trigger, followed by a response or action.

If x happens (trigger) => then y happens (response)
You hear your name (trigger) => you answer (response)

An example would be going to the fridge to eat something even though you are not hungry. The trigger would be going towards, and opening, the fridge.

Words are, of course, the most powerful drug used by mankind
– Rudyard Kipling

The old response would be to take something and eat it. The new post-hypnotic suggestion might be to immediately stop, take a deep breath and ask yourself if you really need to eat this now. Or to make the feel of the fridge door on your hand, or the noise of it opening, a trigger to remind yourself of the resolution you made to eat only when you are truly hungry.

Another example would be for exam nerves. The post-hypnotic trigger is entering the exam room; the suggestion could be, *"As you see the clock on the wall, you imagine the spring unwinding in the clock as all your stress and concerns unwind, as you drop your shoulders, take a deep breath and, feeling relaxed and calm, find your seat."*

Post-hypnotic suggestions are the main tools of hypnosis which bring about desired changes at some point in the future. They are specifically beneficial when using hypnosis to prepare for an actual event, such as taking a driving test, doing a presentation, or preparing for childbirth.

A mum's experience

"I awoke in bed as my waters broke at 2.45 a.m.; I announced the news to my husband and we calmly packed up the car – including the Birth Preparation and the Relaxing Birth Music track. I did not feel any pain throughout the journey. Upon arrival I was told I was 2–3 cm dilated. The nurse offered to place an IV in my arm when she took blood. I declined. Then they monitored the baby's heart and my contractions, although I didn't feel them at this point. Within an hour the contractions became more intense, and by 7 a.m. I was 5–6 cm dilated.

We played the Relaxing Birth Music CD in the room and I breathed and swayed through the waves of intensity. I used the words '3, 2, 1, relax' over and over again. My mind just seemed to know that when I said those words, my whole body would relax. I got back into the birthing pool with the desire to push. The powerful waves pulsated through me and I let out deep, natural grunts. After ten of these incredible pushes, holding onto my husband's hands and the bar on the side of the tub, the baby surfaced and lay peacefully on my chest looking at me. What an empowering, beautiful experience."

Shonda Kohlhoff, Germany

I'm not afraid of storms, for I'm learning to sail my ship
– Louisa May Alcott

For example, if you were using hypnosis to prepare you for a big race, it would be totally impractical and unreasonable to be on the starting line of a race and to ask everyone to suddenly stop while you take yourself into hypnosis. What you really need is to have done all the mental preparation "in advance" so that your body automatically responds in the way you have instructed it to.

As we have seen earlier, your mind stores all your experiences and memories and then holds them until they are needed as references again in the future. By giving your mind a new set of experiences and responses, when the time comes, these are triggered in your mind and you automatically follow the new set of responses. Clinical trials have proven the success of giving these types of suggestions when in hypnosis[2].

Sometimes, following post-hypnotic suggestions will initially take some conscious effort as well; however, after a short period of time, you become less conscious of them, until they become automatic. It is like learning to drive a car – you are initially very aware of which pedal to push, but after a while you no longer even think about it anymore.

Again, as we mentioned before, the more you practise something, the more it becomes instinctive and easy. With post-hypnotic suggestions, the more you hear them, the more your mind takes them on as your own reality. So by "practising" them over and over again, when you then encounter the trigger for real, your mind is quick and instinctive at producing the desired response.

Remember, the mind does not know the difference between things that you have imagined and things that are real.

Dr. Maltz writes that:

> Experimental and clinical psychologists have proved beyond a shadow of a doubt that the human nervous system cannot tell the difference between an 'actual' experience and an experience imagined vividly and in detail.[3]

As you read earlier, you often have the same physiological response to pretend or imagined danger, e.g. a horror film, as you have to real danger. Watching a horror film is not real – you are simply sitting in your living room watching an electronic box with thousands of tiny coloured dots. However, the image that is imprinted in your mind is real and so your body kicks off an adrenalin-rush response.

The greatest danger for most of us is not that our aim is too high and we miss it, but that it is too low and we reach it – Michelangelo

The impact that this can have in a negative way is obvious, so just imagine the benefits and potential if you used this in a positive way. By creating your own "films" showing the positive kind of response that you want, you are more likely to get the same response when the film becomes a reality.

One note of caution: no matter how wonderful the suggestions are, if the person is not really motivated and committed to making the change, then they will not work. The conscious mind can still override post-hypnotic suggestions if the will to change is not there.

Triggers

As we have already seen, the mind makes associations of cause and effect based on our past experiences. We all have triggers (specific stimuli which influence or create a way of feeling or thinking). Triggers occur naturally all the time – when you hear the phone ring, you automatically go to answer it; if you feel a tap on your shoulder, you turn around; when you hear a favourite song, you feel warm and happy; when you hear the "*der der der*" of the music from the film *Jaws*, a feeling of fear rises. Many of our reactions are created by triggers – previous learnt experiences and responses – and, as ever, the more we respond to a trigger, the more entrenched it becomes.

As we are all extremely good at creating triggers already, this is another technique which is extremely powerful when combined with hypnosis. In hypnosis you can create triggers to help bring about positive feelings and responses post-hypnotically. These triggers can be a word, a touch, or even taking a deep breath, and can become an instruction for your mind and body to produce a response, e.g. deep relaxation, a feeling of calm, a sense of being in control. As it is all done in hypnosis, you are again instructing the subconscious part of the mind, and so it is more likely to be imprinted.

This trigger can then be used at any time in the future. As the trigger occurs, the subconscious brings about the feelings and responses that are associated with the trigger. This is extremely beneficial for helping with anxiety, habits, pain management and stress management.

> *Did you know?*
>
> The most famous use of triggers or stimulus response was developed by Pavlov. Each time he fed his dogs he would ring a bell. The dogs soon began to associate the sound (trigger) of the bell with food and would salivate on hearing the bell, even when no food was given.

> *Aerodynamically the bumblebee shouldn't be able to fly, but the bumblebee doesn't know that so it goes on flying anyway – Mary Kay Ash*

"Letting go" exercises

In order to achieve much of the desired change it is often beneficial for there to be an element of "letting go" of old habits, fears, beliefs and patterns of thinking. When asked what keeps us in the pattern of doing things, if we are really honest with ourselves we can usually identify some of the reasons, for example, comfort, sympathy, security, social acceptance. If you ask someone to simply stop doing those things at a conscious level, it is extremely difficult and often impossible, as the old habits and patterns have stayed there for a reason – predominantly to protect us from negative reactions, thoughts and feelings.

If a person is really ready to move on and no longer wants the old ways to rule their life now, then taking them through a "letting go" exercise in hypnosis can produce excellent results. Because you are talking directly to the subconscious, you can access the part of the mind which is normally under lock and key and then allow it to be acknowledged, thanked for its part and then released. It is also useful to then suggest to the subconscious that it replace the old way with one that is more beneficial and useful to the person today.

"Letting go" exercises are usually done through the use of metaphor or storytelling to encourage the person to become aware of any issues before letting them go (see step 3). This is particularly useful for people holding onto unhelpful or unnecessary fears when preparing for birth.

Future pacing

The mind can be a very literal thing. The images we have of ourselves and our beliefs about the way we respond tend to be what happens in reality. The more we see ourselves as overweight, forgetful, self-conscious, unsuccessful, etc, the more we tend to live out the reality. As a result, many of our thoughts become a self-fulfilling prophecy.

Another powerful technique you can use in hypnotherapy to help create new images for yourself is called future pacing. It is a technique in which you imagine, see or feel what it will be like at some point in the future to "be" the person you want to be or to achieve the outcome you want.

When in hypnosis, your mind can be wonderfully vivid in creating images and feelings, so, with any issue that you wish to address, spend time in hypnosis imagining what it will be like, how it will feel, what you will see, and what others will say when you have achieved your outcome – see yourself on the beach being the shape and size that pleases you; see, feel, and

Enthusiasm is the best protection in any situation. Wholeheartedness is contagious.
Give yourself, if you wish to get others – David Seabury

hear yourself making that entertaining and inter-esting speech, hearing the applause, seeing the smiling faces; see, feel, and hear what it will be like to pass your driving test. Be as vivid as you can, and really notice all the details – the smile on your face, the feeling of pride, the congratulations from those around you, the sense of achievement. Make all the sounds, colours, images and details as rich and vivid as possible.

By creating the images, feelings and thoughts in your mind, you are giving yourself a new direction to move towards, giving yourself something "real" and more positive to work towards. Instead of accepting and sticking with the old negative image, the brain is more likely to lead you in the direction of your imagined "future self". This technique is used frequently by top sportsmen such as golfers, who always visualise themselves making the perfect shot before they have even picked up the club.

Did you know?

Future-pacing techniques are used by professionals in all fields of life:

– athletes use it to see, feel and experience themselves winning the race;

– performers use it to see, feel and experience themselves performing successfully in front of an audience;

– even students use it to see, feel or experience themselves sitting the exam, feeling relaxed, calm and confident.

A study by Edmund Jacobson showed that visualising an activity produced a small, but measurable, reaction in the muscles[4]. So, by doing a mental rehearsal of how you would like to respond in future, you are actually implanting a learned memory of a successful action. You are also informing your subconscious mind of what you expect it to achieve.

Again, seeing yourself being successful in the future is far easier in a state of hypnosis. Because you are bypassing the conscious mind, you are not analysing or criticising each image to see how, where, why or when it fits into your preconceived idea of how life should be.

Time distortion

When someone is in hypnosis, their awareness of time can become quite distorted. Time is "man made" – it only exists insofar as we have devised a way to measure the passing of time. As a result, when you are not using the analytical part of your mind, time becomes irrelevant and people often find it difficult to accurately assess how long they have been in hypnosis for.

Appreciation can make a day – even change a life. Your willingness to put it into words is all that is necessary – Margaret Cousins

As a result, you can actually promote this sense of time distortion using post-hypnotic suggestions. This can be very useful when people are travelling, would prefer time to go quickly or are waiting for news such as test results. It is also particularly useful in childbirth as a way for the mother to be unaware of the time, so that her perception is one of having all the time she needs to feel wonderfully relaxed and refreshed between contractions, and the time of each contraction feels as if it is just a few seconds.

A great example of using time distortion was highlighted on one of our courses, when a couple came with their young baby to talk to the prospective parents about their birth experience. The mother was seated on a chair in front of the father, holding her baby. She was telling her version of the birth, saying how she was amazed that each contraction only lasted twenty seconds. Behind her, the father was looking surprised, shaking his head and mouthing the words, "No, they were not."

What had happened was that the mother's perception of time had been so distorted that she really felt as if each contraction was just a few seconds. She had built this time distortion into her hypnosis programme so that her mind was "trained" to experience each contraction

A mum's experience

"I had a wonderful birth experience, which I believe is solely down to the fact that the birth preparation CD removed all fear and anxiety. I was in labour for just over six hours (this was my first baby) and delivered without pain relief. Throughout the labour and birth I felt totally calm and surprisingly I did not feel that I was pushing. Rather, my body seemed to do the work so that I felt my baby being pulled out with each contraction.

I felt that the time in-between each contraction was indeed longer than the Contractions and this time was euphoric. The midwife continually commented on and invited others to come to observe my calm and relaxed demeanour.

Thank you for giving me the means to birth my baby in such a positive and memorable way."

Carol Gregson, UK

I want to be all that I am capable of becoming – Katherine Mansfield

as "just a few seconds". During the birth, she was in a relaxed state with little interference from her mind, so her birthing brain just went with the flow and her perception was what counted.

Exit - Coming out of Hypnosis

Bringing someone out of hypnosis has to be done gently and carefully. If a person has been very relaxed and in a deep hypnotic state, then they need to have time to be able to "come back to normal".

There are five steps to bringing oneself out of hypnosis which are marked by counting from 1 to 5:

1. Restore sensations to their true perspective. You have full co-ordination, flexibility and control throughout your entire body; any feelings of lightness or heaviness return to their true perspective.
2. Restore all sounds to their true perspective.
3. Place yourself back in the room, being aware of what is on your left and your right, above and below you.
4. Begin to come up, bringing with you and keeping all the benefits of this experience.
5. Eyes open and wide awake.

---

[1] Benson, H., 1976, *The Relaxation Response*, New York, Avon Books.

[2] Alman, B. M. & Carney, R. E., "Consequences of Direct and Indirect Suggestion on Success of Post-hypnotic Behaviour", *American Journal of Clinical Hypnosis*, Vol. 23 1080.

[3] Maltz, M., 1960, *Psycho Cybernetics: A New Way to Get More Living Out of Life*, Prentice Hall.

[4] Thomas, C. C., 1967, *Biology of Emotions*, Springfield, Illinois.

Nothing in life is so hard that you can't make it easier by the way you take it
– Ellen Glasgow

A mum's experience

"The birth of my son Angus has been an amazing journey. The first steps in my journey involved me making a big shift in my thinking about birth. This was helped by my sister's and friend's positive experiences of birth and then by a course my husband and I undertook with Natal Hypnotherapy. This course helped us learn how a woman's body is made to give birth; the emotional phases a woman goes through when giving birth; techniques for working with my body while it gives birth; and, above all, the importance of mentally getting out the way and allowing my body to do its job.

On 24 April, I woke at 3 a.m. to the dawn chorus, feeling a bit peculiar. I soon realised Angus was on his way. I lay in the quiet stillness of my room, feeling the gentle tightenings of my uterus. After an hour or so I woke Michael and together we lay chatting, listening to the day awake ... full of excitement and anticipation.

We called my doula, Maggie, and awaited her arrival. I rested in bed, listening to music. By the time Maggie arrived I'd got a little caught up with timings! She took away my watch and suggested I come downstairs which helped me disengage my mind and just get on with being excited about the day ahead .

Gradually, though, I had to concentrate more deeply on my breathing and started to try out different positions. I remember the birth had reached a more serious point when I got off my gym ball and leant over it, rocking gently. Understanding that this was the next natural phase of the birth helped me to focus on ways I could help my body – for me, this involved deep breathing and changing positions frequently. I constantly kept telling myself, too, 'Allow your body to do its job.'

I had decided to give myself plenty of time to get to the hospital. On the journey, my husband recounted a special day we'd spent together, which I visualised. We also said, '3, 2, 1, relax, Emma', a trigger for my brain to let go and relax. I felt myself breathe deeply as I uttered these words.

On reaching the hospital, we realised we'd forgotten our hospital notes. Michael had to go back to get them. At this point I either lost my focus or reached the self-doubt phase I'd learnt about. To my relief, Maggie allowed me to hang on to her and took me through a visualisation which helped calm me. When Michael *returned, I felt I could get down to business. As a complete surprise to me, I stood up and began to stamp my feet and say very loudly, "Come, Angus, come", "Come, baby, come", "Come beautiful boy". It felt so empowering.*

When I reached the delivery room I leant on the window sill and continued with the stamping and was soon shouting. I think the whole hospital knew his name by the time I'd finished! The next hour I experienced more as 10 minutes and remember it as moments in time: staring at Michael's face; Maggie and Michael encouraging me to breathe down; Maggie's relaxation music. It felt quite supernatural and above all, my body felt in control. The midwife said that when I felt to push to start panting. I found this a bit confusing as I started asking myself questions: How hard should I push? When? In retrospect I never felt a desire to push, just an amazing bearing down that my body was in charge of, not me...To my delight, when Angus's head and arms had emerged, the midwife asked if I wanted to deliver him. Instinctively I reached down and pulled him up to me. I was lying on a beanbag and it felt safe to be close to the ground with this little life. Angus breathed his first breath and took his first cry. What an amazing and perfect sound.

The time after this was one of immense peace, calm and joy. Michael and I just sat in complete amazement, cradling our son, examining every part of him. We didn't feel rushed but relaxed in an atmosphere of joy and peace.

I was particularly amazed how great I felt so soon after giving birth. I was up and about chatting, eating toast, marvelling at my son. I felt ready to get on with looking after him and felt well and elated. The last hour or so my body worked hard, but it wasn't unlike running up a steep, steep hill at the end of a long run. But unlike a run, my body was in charge of making my uterus work hard, not me, in a similar way to my heart beating with or without my help. I wasn't exhausted at this last stage either, having spent the day managing the contractions peacefully and in a relaxed atmosphere at home.

Angus's birth has taught me a great deal: the importance of giving my body and mind good, positive images and thoughts, nutritious food, adequate sleep and ways to relax. In doing so, I feel more able (most of the time at least!) to manage more challenging situations in life...Above all, I am just so happy that the first hours of Angus' life were so beautiful and that I was happy, well and overjoyed to see him."

Emma Trim, UK

Part 3

Chapter 9 – Five steps to a better birth

Now that you have a better understanding of:

- the instinctive process of giving birth;
- how your body works best during birth;
- how your mind works;
- and what Natal Hypnotherapy is and how it can help,

it is time to turn towards the practical tools and techniques that will help you have a more instinctive and empowering birth experience.

By following Natal Hypnotherapy's five steps, you will prepare yourself positively and effectively for birth.

1. Overcome fear

2. Learn ways to deal with pain

3. Know you can do it

4. Acquire practical skills

5. Prepare your birth partner

Outcome:

Reduced need for drugs or intervention

More likely to have a positive birth

Relaxed, calm mother and birth partner

Increased bonding with your baby

Calm, alert baby

Step 1 – Overcome fear

"Hopes and fears" exercise

The first and most important step to overcoming any fears is to acknowledge and face them head on. Bringing them out into the open, writing them down, and talking about them either on a course or to someone you are close to is a huge step forward. This is especially the case for birth partners, who may never have had the opportunity to speak up in a safe, supported environment about what worries them.

By bringing your fears up to the surface now, they will not become the lurking "tiger" in the shadows, ready to pounce once you are in the vulnerable state of giving birth. As you will soon realise, fears are simply thoughts. They are not concrete activities that will take place for definite: they are simply thoughts derived from the sum of your previous experiences. And,

A mum's experience

"I _was_ one of those women who, from the age of seven, was totally terrified of the thought of giving birth. Thankfully, I found out about Natal Hypnotherapy. Miraculously, I felt I was able to completely overcome my fears and so went into the birth feeling calm and prepared, not petrified and scared.

On the day, I went into a totally hypnotic world of peace and calm – I closed my eyes throughout, breathed deeply at each contraction and was sprayed with cool water and had a flannel on my forehead. My sister, who is a midwife, was present and couldn't believe her sister was being so calm, relaxed and in control throughout the whole labour. I can honestly say I _enjoyed_ – yes, enjoyed – the birth with the aid of these tools.

I cannot thank you enough – 28 years of worry (such wasted energy) ending in such a wonderful birth."

Elizabeth McGowan, UK

A baby will make love stronger, days shorter, nights longer, bankroll smaller, home happier, clothes shabbier, the past forgotten, and the future worth living for
– Author unknown

as with any thought, we can accept them, let them go and change them for ones that are more useful and beneficial.

How to do it yourself

Turn back to the beginning of the book, where you completed your pregnancy and birth profile. Read through the fears and concerns that you had and add to them if you feel anything has changed.

Now take some post-it notes or a pad of paper and begin by writing down one fear or concern on each post-it note. Be completely open to your thoughts and make a note of anything that comes to mind. It does not matter how silly or small it may seem – if your subconscious has brought it to your attention, then pay attention!

Once you have written them all down, stick them in the back of this book. Simply by writing them down, you have started the process of letting them go. Again, as you go through your pregnancy, any concerns that arise, write them down and add them to the back of the book. You can then go on to the "letting go" exercises and focus on either one at a time or all of them in one go.

A mum's experience

"I was quite fearful of giving birth, which led me to using the Natal Hypnotherapy.
It was only when I listened to the track that I realised just how afraid I was. I would often cry after listening because of all the horror stories I'd heard from other people and the uncertainty of how things would turn out for me. Through listening to the tracks, I realised I didn't have to be afraid: my body is designed to give birth and I can do it.

They gave me confidence in myself and my body. So, during labour, I told myself to shut down the thinking part of my brain, relax and let my body get on with it, making sure that I was breathing deeply. My partner gave me a back massage during contractions as well, which helped. Overall, I'd say my birth experience was a positive one and the birth preparation track really helped me a lot to prepare for it."

Jane Naysmith, UK

There is no friendship, no love, like that of a mother for her child
– Henry Ward Beecher

Once you have done this a few times, listened to the CDs or attended a course, go back to your post-It notes. If there are any fears that you feel fit in the following categories, then you can take them out, tear them up and throw them away:

1. They no longer worry you.
2. You realise that there is nothing you can do about it now, so you will simply no longer let it take any of your energy or thought.
3. You are still concerned, but you are going to plan ways to understand what you can do so that it no longer worries you.

"Letting go" exercise

This is one of the most powerful elements to Natal Hypnotherapy, as it allows you to access any fears in your subconscious and then give yourself permission to let them go. As the exercises that couples do on the course are done in hypnosis, their subconscious is very open and honest about their fears. As a result, many couples may find that fears they had not thought were of

A mum's experience

"After a really terrible experience with my first son, I was determined to find a different way when I got pregnant this time. My biggest fear came from the old memories, which still gave me nightmares. I felt sure that the same would happen again. When I did the Natal Hypnotherapy course, there were two things which really stood out.

The first was that I can now see why and when things started to go wrong last time – if only I had known all of that first time round. Secondly, the "letting go" exercises were so powerful. I actually felt the bad memories leave my mind – it was surreal. I was able to completely let go of them and they did not come back. The nightmares stopped, and with all the other techniques I had learnt I spent the rest of my pregnancy looking forward to the birth and not dreading it.

Baby Joshua was born peacefully and calmly in hospital after six hours of labour. None of the old fears came back and I was amazed at how calm, focused and relaxed I was. I wish every woman had access to these techniques. Thank you."

Jennifer Radley, UK

Think of stretch marks as pregnancy service stripes – Joyce Armor

any importance came up, or even that ones they had not consciously been aware of came to the forefront.

This "letting go" can be very liberating as you begin to realise that fear is nothing but an emotion – it is not "real", "tangible" or permanent – and that many fears do not serve a beneficial purpose.

Once you realise that worrying about something is a huge waste of energy and does nothing but focus on the negative, you can put your fears behind you and move forward in a more positive, beneficial away.

> *Did you know?*
> Pampering yourself means pampering your baby. Don't feel selfish if you need to rest or treat yourself to organic food or healthy fruit smoothies.

How to do it yourself

There are lots of ways to let go of fears. You can take the post-it notes that you have written and scrunch them up and put them in the bin, or better still throw them into a fire. You can take each fear and tie it to a helium balloon and watch as they float up into the sky. You can imagine that a small candle represents a fear and then watch as it slowly melts away. You can imagine that small twigs or leaves represent your fears and then watch as they float away down a river.

All of these can be done in reality, but they can also be done in hypnosis using visualisation or your imagination. Before you start, think of a metaphor for letting go – maybe sending fears off on clouds, maybe throwing them down a well, or maybe seeing them floating off down a stream. Then, when you are ready, take yourself into a nicely relaxed state by focusing on your breathing and then on relaxing each part of your body. Use the pages at the end of this book to write down ones that appeal to you.

Spend a few moments visualising something or somewhere calm and relaxing – maybe a beach, maybe a summer garden, maybe a happy memory. When you feel at ease and relaxed, ask your subconscious to bring one of your fears to your attention. Spend a moment thinking about it, accepting it, even thanking it for the purpose it has served up until now. Ask your subconscious to hold onto any positive learning the fear may have given you and to let go of any negative or unhelpful feelings.

> *It is not until you become a mother that your judgment slowly turns to compassion and understanding – Erma Bombeck*

Then, when you are ready, let it go by whatever means you feel comfortable with. Allow the fear to float, drift, or sink away so that it is no longer a part of you, no longer able to hold you back. As it goes further from you, any anxiety, any negative thoughts connected with the fear, become less and less as you become more and more at ease, lighter, calmer.

You can then repeat this process to deal with other fears or concerns.

This is an exercise you can do at any time, and even during the birth. If at any time you have a fear or concern, spend a few moments acknowledging it and then letting it go. This will free your mind and body to get back to the business of birthing and to trusting that your body is doing all it needs to do.

Remember to take this book and your notes with you so that your birth partner can have it as a prompt to use if he or she notices that you are having any concerns or are tensing up in any way.

A mum's experience

"At 4.25 a.m. we welcomed our son Gilli, born at home on Monday, 7 April – his father's birthday! The actual due date. Weighing 7 lbs 1 oz. A true gift from above!

We went to bed around 10 p.m., did some Chi Quong, and I dabbed a little clary sage and rose oil on my dressing gown. At 11.25 p.m., bang! The first contraction, and it was pretty serious. I was shaking and felt like I went into shock. This was it! We must have missed the 'excitement phase' and not realised I was in labour. I'd been getting what I thought were strong Braxton Hicks the whole day and saw each one as an opportunity to breathe deeply and practise the techniques. We phoned for the midwife about twenty minutes later, when contractions were around three minutes apart.

It was intense (to say the least), but with huge help from my husband, Steve (I would not let him leave my side!), I was able to 'turn down' each contraction, so I felt each one for about twenty seconds instead of the full length. We lay on our bed facing each other, and as each contraction came I said 'COMFORT' and Steve

Mother love is the fuel that enables a normal human being to do the impossible
– Marion C. Garretty

would count down slowly, 10–9–8 ... turning down the intensity to zero. After a second (where is she!?!) call from Steve, the midwife arrived around 30–45 minutes later.

She was perfect, as she pretty much sat at the end of our bed and left us to it. Around 1.30 a.m. a second midwife arrived and we decided to see how much I had dilated. 7 cm. 'Brilliant,' we all thought, baby will be here soon! But after a few hours, things had slowed down. I got tired and entered the 'self-doubt phase'.

Fortunately, thanks to the Natal Hypnotherapy course, I knew exactly what was happening. I was saying, 'I can't do this,' but I was also saying, 'Oh no, this is the self-doubt phase. I know I can do it, but I feel like I can't.' It was actually quite funny.

Throughout the labour I tried a few different positions – kneeling on the floor, sat on the loo, kneeling on the bed – and I had a warm bath, but for the most part lying on my left side facing Steve worked for me.

He kept me focused and turned the imaginary dial with his hand. We even managed a giggle when at one point I told him he was turning the dial the wrong way! When it was time to push I sat up in our bed. The thought of pushing made me suddenly awake and renewed with energy! This part probably took between 15 and 20 minutes. With lots of encouragement from the midwives, out he popped. We woke our two kids, aged 12 and 10 (as they had requested), seconds after he was born and they watched as Steve cut the cord.

My big fear was that I would scream the house down with pain and embarrass myself, but it didn't happen. Sometimes I moaned, sometimes just deep breathing and counting out loud. No pain relief and an ever-so-tiny tear. It was just wonderful to deliver at home in our bed. And the best part was all of us being able to huddle together moments after he was born. Nobody had to leave. Beautiful.

Thank you to the Natal Hypnotherapy course for giving us the confidence to do it! And of course to the midwives and my husband Steve – I could not have done it without you!"

Shirley Gordon, UK

Step 2 – Learn ways to deal with pain

Unlike most pain that is associated with injury, illness or stress, the sensations of labour are the result of a normal, healthy bodily function. By allowing your body to do its job, and by accepting and recognising the sensations of each contraction as productive and positive, you can help reduce the pain to a more manageable level.

Deep physical relaxation and beneficial breathing

A vitally important step towards reducing pain during childbirth is to learn how to breathe deeply and relax your body to such a point that there is no tension in your muscles.

A mum's experience

"I would like to share my positive feedback on the birth of my baby boy, Sacha, thanks to Natal Hypnotherapy. I listened to the tracks lots of times and felt mentally prepared and very calm before the birth. I had written down some key words and sentences from the track, and, as soon as labour started, all the important key words came back. I had a very long labour but managed throughout with breathing techniques and by remaining focused and relaxed. When the contractions were at their peak, I managed to keep my body very relaxed.

There was no tension at all, and I believe this is the reason why I did not feel any pain. I did feel the intensity of the contractions – it was almost like an out-of-body experience – but at no stage did I scream out of pain.

I also believe the reason why I managed to stay calm is because my husband was at home and the labour ward I was in was very quiet, so I could completely focus and work with my body without any distractions. I fully recommend the Natal Hypnotherapy. The birth of my baby was a very positive experience and not at all traumatic."

Nathalie Pajot, France

A woman has two smiles that an angel might envy: the smile that accepts a lover before words are uttered, and the smile that lights on the first-born babe, and assures it of a mother's love – Thomas C. Haliburton

By learning how to do this during pregnancy using hypnosis, post-hypnotic suggestions and triggers, you will condition your body to go totally limp during a contraction.

This will help:

- to channel all your excess energy to your uterus

- your blood pressure to stay low

- your breathing to be more effective

- your baby to receive plenty of oxygen

- the muscles of the uterus to have no "competition" from tension in your other muscles

- to ensure that you stay calm, focused and relaxed

> **Did you know?**
>
> In 1652, Philip Barrough wrote in his book *The Method of Physick* that if women were encouraged to breathe and relax their pelvic region, it would ease the discomfort of birth.

As we have already seen, deep breathing and relaxation are natural components of hypnosis, and the more you practise this during your pregnancy, the more natural and instinctive it will be during the birth.

The most important points to remember, no matter what else you do, are to:

1. Breathe slowly, rhythmically and deeply, imagining that each breath goes all the way down to your baby.

2. During contractions, make sure that all the muscles in your body are as relaxed as possible, so channelling all your energy to your uterus.

Breathing techniques

You have been breathing all your life, and by now should be quite good at it!

When it comes to giving birth, you do not need to learn any complicated or altered breathing patterns. I do not advocate or teach any special ways of breathing, as I feel that this can add more "consciousness" to giving birth, so taking you away from your primal instincts. The more you can follow what your body is asking of you, the more likely you are to breathe effectively.

> *At the end of the day, a loving family should find everything forgivable*
> *– Mark V. Olsen and Will Scheffer*

There are only two things that you need to know about breathing. The first is to breathe down to your abdomen or down to your baby, and the second is to breathe rhythmically and slowly.

Abdominal breathing

Throughout the birthing process, the more you breathe steadily, evenly and deeply – breathing down to your tummy, feeling it rise and expand – the better it will be for you and your baby. This kind of breathing is totally natural and normal when you are in a relaxed state.

The only difference during the birthing process is that you become very focused on your breathing: you listen to it and observe it so that you can consciously, deliberately ensure it is calm, rhythmic and deep.

This kind of breathing is synonymous with relaxation, and, as you are aware, relaxation is THE KEY to a comfortable birth experience. By listening to your breathing, and keeping it steady, rhythmical and deep, you keep tension away – with no tension, the uterus can do its job far more effectively.

As well as the emotionally and mentally calming effects of abdominal breathing, you will benefit physically in many ways:

- By expanding your abdomen as well as your lungs, you give the vertical muscles of the uterus more room to reach down and pull up the circular muscles.

- Your blood pressure remains at a healthy level.

- You increase the level of oxygen to your uterine muscles and to your baby.

- You increase the level of oxytocin (hormone responsible for regulating contractions).

- This increases the level of prostaglandin (the hormone which softens the cervix) and relaxin (hormone for stretching the perineum).

- This increases the level of endorphins (the hormone that dulls the sensations in the part of the brain which registers pain).

The family is one of nature's masterpieces – George Santayana

Breathing exercises

By listening to a Natal Hypnotherapy CD, MP3 or attending a course, you will learn all you need to know about breathing. As you will be practising your own method of breathing repeatedly before the birth of your baby, and as it is done in association with the birth visualisation, your subconscious mind becomes imprinted with your breathing patterns and is then able to recreate them during the birth.

During your pregnancy, it is useful to practise slow, rhythmic breathing and for your partner to be aware of your breathing patterns, so that they can recognise any changes to those patterns during the labour. A change in your breathing pattern during the birth can indicate rises in adrenalin or tension, which are best avoided.

How to do it yourself

Get yourself in a comfortable position and turn off all distractions.

If you are with your partner, ask them to sit with their back resting against a wall and with their knees apart, forming a contour chair for you to relax into. Sit between their knees, resting back against their chest. Ask your partner to reach their arms around you so that their hands gently rest on your tummy, with their fingers facing down to your pelvis. They will need to pay particular attention to the feeling of your tummy rising and falling, being aware of the pace of your breathing.

Mum: Lie back and relax into your partner's arms. Close your eyes and begin by focusing your thoughts on your breathing.

With each breath in, think of sending your breath way down into your lower tummy or to where your baby lies. Imagine that the muscles of your abdomen are extremely relaxed. The abdomen will naturally expand outward, so you do not need to push your tummy out or try to hold it. Listen to the sound of your breathing, and keep it calm, steady, rhythmical.

It is important to note that breathing deeply does not mean taking a huge, deep breath – it is simply a breath, which goes deeper down to your abdomen. By listening to your breathing, you stay in the moment, making it impossible to breathe too quickly, to hold your breath or to breathe shallowly, which can lead to hyperventilation.

Other things may change us, but we start and end with the family
– Anthony Brandt

After a few moments, discuss with each other:

What did you notice about the pace of your breathing?

How did it differ from your partner?

Did you naturally get in-sync, or were your breathing rates very different?

Breathing exercise – Matching and pacing breathing

Partners: During labour, one of the key things to be looking out for is if there is any change in her breathing patterns. This can indicate a degree of anxiety, tension or fear. If this were to happen, one of the quickest and most effective ways to help her relax is to slow down and exaggerate your own breathing pattern so that she will naturally get back in-sync with you.

You can practise this using the following exercise:

Mum: Sitting in the same position as before, begin breathing normally.

Partner: Sitting in the same position, concentrate on matching your breathing to hers. This can be a little strange and feel a bit forced, as pregnant women tend to breathe more slowly. Once you are both in the same rhythm, it is important for the birth partner to keep this rhythm throughout the exercise.

Mum: After a short while, consciously change your breathing to a shallower, faster pace. Try to keep this up as long as possible, until you really have had enough and want to get back to your deep breathing.

Partner: Once you notice the change in her breathing, exaggerate your slow, deep breathing with the aim of encouraging her to go back to the deep breathing.

After a few moments, discuss with each other:

How did it feel when you were in sync?

How did it feel when you were not in sync?

How easy was it for the mum to stay breathing quickly?

How long did it last?

How did it feel when you went back to breathing together?

This is a useful exercise for the birth, as, if the partner notices that the mum's breathing has become faster and shallower, then simply doing loud, slow, deep breaths will remind her, in a non-verbal way, to get back into a quiet, deep rhythm.

A man's work is from sun to sun, but a mother's work is never done –
Author unknown

Breathing exercise – Horse breathing

This may sound a bit odd, but it is a great exercise to help loosen and relax all the muscles in the jaw, which, in turn, will relax the muscles in the birth canal and perineum.

Allow your lips to become really loose and floppy, then blow air out, making your lips gently vibrate. This will naturally relax your jaw and neck and release tension in general. We often naturally do this when we feel relieved or want to relax.

It is useful to remember to do this at intervals during the birth, especially as your baby is close to being born.

Extra tip: This is a great exercise to do if you are feeling constipated, as it can help relax all The relevant muscles!

Did you know?
Aymara women of South America carry their babies with them at all times and sleep with them until they are at least two years old.

Relaxation techniques

An untrained mother would find it very hard, if not impossible, to suddenly relax during labour. Well-meaning midwives often say, "try and relax". The mother bravely "tries" by making her body appear still and quiet, but that is very different from genuinely letting go of all the tension in her body.

Relaxation sounds easy, but in fact it is something that needs practice in order to achieve the kind of deep relaxation needed for the birth. Relaxation is your foundation – everything else depends on it, everything builds on it. If you are tense during a contraction, the uterus has to work twice as hard to do the same amount of work, as the other muscles are straining against the uterus, making it more painful.

Learning how to relax at will is a skill.

The purpose is to ensure that your body stays totally limp, allowing your birthing muscles to work unimpeded by other bodily tensions. This may sound easy, but, though it is simple, it is not easy, and initially it may take all your concentration to keep your whole body limp and free of tension. Your ability to relax during contractions will directly correlate to your degree of comfort.

It's so good to know that wherever you are, a Mom is with you in spirit and in love
– Author unknown

According to Johnston in one of the early midwifery textbooks:

> *The woman who can relax has a shorter and easier first stage, and in the second stage her pelvic floor will offer less resistance.*

To become skilful at relaxing, you have to become skilful at noticing tension and then releasing it. Once you recognise it, you can release it. It is not like going to sleep, where you just wait for your body to relax – this is something that you do with intention.

How to do it yourself

In your daily routine, regularly check to see if there is any tension in your body – drop your shoulders, relax your hands, relax your back. You will be amazed at how often we hold tension in our body. If you feel any tension rising in your body, take a deep breath, a long exhale, and actively relax that part of your body. By doing this several times a day, you will soon recognise when your body feels tense and when it is relaxed.

Using hypnosis for relaxation

Using hypnosis is such a wonderful way of learning relaxation, as the more you do it, the easier it becomes, and, unlike learning other new skills, it is wonderfully enjoyable and relaxing from the outset. It is simply a matter of lying back, closing your eyes and relaxing your body. There are many different techniques for achieving a relaxed state and many different types of visualisations which help you achieve this.

One of the most common is called a 'fractional relaxation'. This involves focusing on different parts of your body and gradually releasing tension in each area. You can use colours to show a change from tension to relaxation as you start at the top of your head and gradually move down to your face, your neck, your shoulders, your back, and so on. This is especially useful if you are experiencing any discomfort in any part of your body, such as your pelvis or back, as you can linger on that area, imagining that you are releasing all discomfort, filling that area with warmth, comfort and a sense of calm.

As you move down across your stomach, you can spend some time focusing on your baby. Imagine your baby smiling and moving freely, seeing your baby in your mind's eye being calm, at ease and enjoying this relaxation as much as you do. As you continue down your body, you

> *No matter how old a mother is, she watches her middle-aged children for signs of improvement – Florida Scott-Maxwell*

may experience a feeling of heaviness, lightness or tingling – that is normal, and a sign that your body is really relaxing and letting go.

A second and very powerful way of relaxing the body is using a form of progression through counting or a sense of movement. You may like to imagine that you are at the top of a safe, wide staircase with a firm handrail and ten steps ahead of you. Imagine that as you slowly and carefully go down each stair, you become more and more relaxed, letting all your muscles become more and more limp, soft, at ease. As you count down each step, your body becomes progressively heavier, softer and more relaxed, so that, by the time you get to one, you are fully relaxed and at ease.

This technique is also commonly used during the birth by counting through a contraction.

Once you have practised this several times, it gets easier and easier, and sometimes just counting down itself will get you into that relaxed state.

Another technique which is used a great deal in hypnosis is to actively create a response or association to an event or trigger. As you read earlier, everything we do has a cause and an effect.

Remember the x => y?

Every action has a reaction, many of which are instinctive – e.g., you feel heat or pain so you move your hand away, you hear your name so you answer. In the same way, it is easy to create your own "triggers and responses" to help you achieve a resource state, or a way of feeling "on command".

For example, you can tell your subconscious that every time you feel a hand on your shoulder or a light touch on your forehead (trigger), your body will respond by becoming wonderfully relaxed and calm (response). The more you do this, the more that new response is embedded, and the more your subconscious takes it on as your new pattern or way of doing things.

However, it is important to remember that you need to do this over and over again. When you get a new ring on your mobile phone, in the beginning you often ignore it, as you do not think it is your phone; however, over time, you remember, as you have made the subconscious association, and soon you automatically reach for it when it rings.

You can use any trigger you like to achieve a deep state of relaxation, to promote calm breathing down to your baby, to relax your shoulders, and so on.

Every beetle is a gazelle in the eyes of its mother - Moorish proverb

It could be:
- Auditory – the use of special words, a phrase such as '3, 2, 1, relax', or a sound;

- Kinaesthetic – a special touch or stroke or feeling;

- Visual – seeing an image in your mind or in reality, such as a photograph or the sight of a baby's toy or item of clothing;

- Olfactory – using familiar and pleasant smells, such as aromatherapy oils.

Use the notes pages at the end of this book to write down your personal triggers and responses. Again, this is another tool for your birth partner to use during the birth, as, by then, simply saying the words or touching your shoulder will bring about the desired response of relaxation and calm.

Another great way of achieving a learnt, triggered response is through music. By listening to the same relaxing music every time you practise your relaxation, breathing and hypnosis, you are making a subconscious association with that music and deep relaxation. Therefore, when you play that music during the birth, it is yet another way for the birthing brain and body to work together to stay deeply calm and relaxed.

You can combine all these triggers so that your partner can string them together to take you into a deeply relaxed state, quickly and easily.

For example:

In a moment, you will hear me say the words '3, 2, 1, relax' and feel my hand on your forehead, and as you do so your body will become more and more relaxed … 3, 2, 1, relax … that's right. And as you feel my hands press down on your shoulders, your muscles soften and release as you let all the tension flow out of your body … on 3, 2, 1, relax … wonderful, and each note of the music you hear is helping you drift down and down into deep, calm relaxation, on 3, 2, 1, relax.

In this short piece, you and your partner will have connected to your visual, auditory and physical senses. By practising over and over again, and by reinforcing the triggers through their hypnosis, many women are able to enter a deeply relaxed state simply by hearing the trigger words '3, 2, 1, relax' or feeling the touch on their forehead or shoulder.

Using these kinds of triggers makes up a significant part of the Natal Hypnotherapy techniques taught at the courses, and couples are taught how to do this to take each other into a deep state of relaxation.

My mother had a slender, small body, but a large heart – a heart so large that everybody's joys found welcome in it, and hospitable accommodation
– Mark Twain

Visualisation

As we have already discussed, the mind is an incredibly powerful tool, through which you can use imagery and visualisation to help reduce stress and pain, as well as to increase health and well-being. As science is recognising this more and more, there are a plethora of research studies looking at the beneficial impact of mental imagery on pain, skin disease, diabetes, breast cancer, arthritis, headaches and severe burns.

It is important to reiterate that just because we use the words "visual" it does not mean that you have to be able to "see" pictures. Many people find it difficult to visualise and so may shy away from following this exercise. It does not matter how you do it – it is more the process. Some people simply hear sounds or feel the experience of being there.

Whichever sense you use the most, and however you experience the world, just go with whichever way feels right for you. However, for the sake of simplicity, I will continue to use the word "visualisation".

A mum's experience

"I was brought up in Cornwall, by the sea, and our house was up on a cliff, with steps going down to the sea. I had used different relaxation methods during my pregnancy, so I was surprised that in labour this imagery just came to me. At the beginning of each contraction, I imagined myself lighting a small tea candle and then walking slowly down each step cut into the cliff, until I reached the shore. I then placed the tea light on the beach and made my way back up the stairs for the end of the contraction. Without being aware of what I was doing, I found that as the labour progressed there were more and more tea lights on the beach, until the whole beach was alight with tiny candles – it was so beautiful and serene.

Even when the contractions became more intense I almost looked forward to each one, as it meant that I would add another light on the beach. When I went through self-doubt, Andy reminded me about the beach (he had hardly said anything up until then) and I was able to get my focus back and carry on. It was very strange, as, towards the end, the imagery changed as I realised that I was actually carrying my baby in my arms as I went down to the beach – a couple of minutes later I felt the urge to push, and our daughter was born shortly after that."

Mandy Jennings, UK

Don't compromise yourself. You are all you've got – Janis Joplin

Using visualisation as part of your birth preparation helps to take you into a deeply relaxed state, which naturally helps to reduce levels of discomfort and helps you mentally switch off from what is happening in your body. By practising visualisation during your pregnancy, it will become second nature and very comforting, so that during the birth your mind is already familiar with, and used to, the process.

In addition, you will be using visualisation as part of your self-hypnosis programme in the next step in this book. However, for this section, it is a tool that you will use in your preparation as well as a comfort measure during the birth itself.

How to do it yourself

Begin by thinking about a special place. This can be any place you have been to that you have really loved: maybe somewhere on holiday, a garden, the mountains or even your own room.

A mum's experience

"After my waters breaking at 33 weeks, I could not have the home water birth that I was hoping for. But I had listened to the MP3s before, so I used the techniques while I went into the delivery suite at the hospital to calm down. I drove myself to hospital and checked in, and I was not anywhere near as scared of the hospital as I thought I would be. Throughout a night of contractions (five minutes apart from start to finish!) I had put all the energy I had into concentrat- ing on the Natal Hypnotherapy techniques and visualisations that I had learned.

I was not 100% sure that I was in labour, as I was expecting much, much worse, and other expectant mothers were making a real noise in the ward! At the eighth hour of contractions, the visualisations were getting difficult as the contractions became stronger, so I asked for a paracetamol. After a visit from the doctor, it was confirmed that I was 8 cm dilated, and I was rushed to delivery. I was so caught up in the visualisations I forgot to ring my husband to tell him I was in labour! After 15 minutes of pushing, Bethany Hannah Leek was born, weighing 5 lbs 8 oz. Thank you for helping me have a very, very positive birth experience!"

Kissi Wilde, UK

Don't fear failure so much that you refuse to try new things. The saddest summary of a life contains three descriptions: could have, might have, and should have
– Louis E. Boone

Anywhere that represents a feeling of calm, relaxation, happiness or peace. You can even make it up or go somewhere you have seen on the TV. It can be real or a complete fairytale.

You may already do this naturally. Unbeknownst to me, I have been doing this all my life.

When I was very young, I used to go to sleep by imagining that I was on a magic carpet flying off to different countries, where I would have amazing adventures. Then, as I got older, I used to imagine I was diving on a coral reef, where I found a secluded cave underwater that was full of beautiful cushions. I could go there in my mind and no one could disturb me.

When I first learnt hypnosis, we were encouraged to come up with a special place, which for me has stayed the same for many years – it is always a beach I went to many years ago on the island of Koh Samet in Thailand. It was exquisitely beautiful. In my many trips there in my mind, I have sometimes been alone and sometimes with my boys or friends.

When I was pregnant with my first son, I had a really moving moment when, during a hypnosis visualisation, I was swimming around in the sea and suddenly realised that my baby was holding onto my shoulders and swimming with me. Since then, I have been there when all my boys are fully grown and even when I am an old woman. To me it is a wonderful safe haven, a sanctuary to go to where I know that other thoughts will not reach me, and where I will always have a deep sense of happiness and calm.

This process does not have to take long – you can stay in this place for a few seconds or several minutes. Once you are used to "going there" you can be there in a split second.

So be creative! Your imagination is limitless. Whatever you choose to visualise or imagine, make your experience as detailed as possible: see it, smell it, taste it, touch it, hear it, and lastly throw in a dose of emotion – love it, cherish it, enjoy it, marvel at it!

As Napoleon Hill said,

> *"Your subconscious mind recognises and acts upon only thoughts which have been well-mixed with emotion or feeling;* and
>
> *You will get no appreciable results until you learn to reach your subconscious mind with thoughts or spoken words which have been well emotionalised with belief.*[1] "

You can use this exercise to create your "special place", which you can go to during the birth, as a way to "step away" from what is happening around you and to focus your thoughts elsewhere.

> *How wonderful it is that nobody need wait a single moment before starting to improve the world – Anne Frank*

Again, use the notes section at the back of this book to write down a description of your special place. This can then be read back to you during the labour. However, remember that, during the birth, you will probably come up with your own visualisations and special place as well.

Bringing it together – with a stimulus!

Once you have created a few of your own triggers, have your own special place and have practised deep relaxation and breathing, this is a useful exercise to show yourself that all this practice and preparation can actually make a difference to your perception and awareness of discomfort.

So, to give your breathing and relaxation a bit of focus, the next exercise will incorporate a stimulus during your practice. It is wonderfully easy to relax and breathe when you are completely comfortable, so this exercise will help you learn how to stay focused while you are experiencing a degree of discomfort.

The stimulus can be a pinch on the arm or inner thigh, or a wrist burn, ideally given by your partner. Whichever you choose, ask your partner to begin slowly and gently and then to build the pressure to a peak at about 20 seconds, tailing off after 40 seconds. This is to simulate the duration of a contraction.

Mum: Get into a comfortable position and begin by getting into your breathing rhythm. When you hear your trigger word or a phrase such as '3, 2, 1, relax', take an even deeper breath and feel your whole body relaxing and letting go even more. You can then continue to focus on your breathing, on visualising your special place or simply on relaxing your body.

Partner: Once you feel that she is relaxed and her breathing has found a steady rhythm, gently put your hand on her shoulder, saying your trigger words. As she hears this, she will sink into even deeper relaxation, allowing her body to go wonderfully limp and relaxed. Then put your hands on her wrist and begin to pinch or twist lightly at first, then increasing in intensity, holding it at around twenty seconds and then slowly releasing after about a minute.

As with anything, the more you practise this exercise, the easier it will be for the mother to simply focus her mind elsewhere, whilst accepting that the sensations on her arm are there for a short while and then are gone.

---

[1] Hill, N., 1987, *Think and Grow Rich*, Ballantine Books.

Fears are like a mirage. It only happens to be there due to our imagination or reflections of possibilities. The nearer we get to it, the more it disappears
– Samuel Adinoyi

A mum's experience

"Having used hypnotherapy and self-hypnosis for a number of years and experienced the sometimes life-changing results, it wasn't a question of if I would use it during my pregnancy and the birth of Danuta, but rather how I could use it. Not only had I never given birth before, but we had our hearts set on a home birth, which sadly my doctor was very negative about, making me feel like I was being selfish and irresponsible.

For me, learning Natal Hypnotherapy turned the whole 'what-if-it-goes-wrong' starting point on its head; it focuses instead on the perfect and unique birthing experience for the individual woman or couple. I loved being able to visualise my birth and spend the weeks leading up to the birth indulging myself in 'rehearsing' the birth over and over again. For me, Christmas is a very special time of year that holds with it feelings of childhood excitement and happiness – just the smell of a mince pie or the sound of carols being sung makes me glow inside, so the fact that our baby was due around this time had all the makings of the best Christmas ever.

Throughout my pregnancy I had spent time listening to a natal hypnosis relaxation CD, which, whilst increasing my bond with our growing baby inside, also helped me tune into my natural instincts as a mother-to-be. In the third trimester, Adam and I attended a Natal Hypnotherapy weekend. This is when we really began to focus our minds on the actual birth and the writing of our own birthing programme. Using emotive language that was very specific to our own personalities, we developed a script that described the perfect birthing experience – how we would feel, how we would react to certain phases or situations, images, sounds and smells that would trigger positive emotional responses. For example:

... the sounds of the music, which are now familiar to me, reinforce my natural feelings of relaxation and calm ...

... looking into the magical Christmas bauble allows me to fall deeper and deeper into a comfortable, peaceful feeling of complete relaxation ...

... with each contraction I visualise my cervix softening and opening slowly, softening and opening gently, smoothly and easily ...

If we wait for the moment when everything, absolutely everything, is ready, we shall never begin – Ivan Turgenev

I would read the birthing programme often, really soaking up the words that meant so much to us, and, once in a relaxed state of self-hypnosis, I would then recall these words, images and feelings to the sounds of music that would accompany us in the birthing experience. The more often I listened, the deeper into my subconscious these associations were going. The Christmas-tree bauble I knew so well, the stocking hung by the fireplace ready for baby's presents, the smell of Christmas spices – all of these factors meant excitement, comfort, happiness, and deeper and deeper confidence to birth our baby safely and naturally.

The due date came and went. As the days ticked by, talk was turning to induction – this is when I felt my most scared, not because of the dangers of letting me go over, but because I just felt baby wasn't ready yet and that he or she would decide when it was time to meet us. Things were happening – we'd had a show and, having had contractions on and off for two weeks, I was already 3 cm dilated. Fourteen days after her official due date, and on the day we were due to go into hospital, baby Danuta decided it was time to join us – and she wasn't hanging about either.

The experience certainly wasn't without pain, and there was no time for birthing music CDs or Christmas spice oils, but I wouldn't change a single moment. Focusing on each contraction took me deep down into the experience, and during the later stages the visualisation of my cervix softening and opening was intensely powerful and effective. Adam was fully involved at all times and helped communicate my feelings to the midwife during contractions, as well as somehow knowing what to say at the right time. We birthed our daughter in our front room, next to the Christmas tree and in front of the open fire and Christmas stockings. Four-and-a-half hours after waking with strong contractions, I was holding Danuta in my arms, crying at the beauty of our perfect baby girl who had ensured that there will always be fireworks on her birthday by being born on a magical New Year's Eve.

With the support and confidence of an amazing partner, an experienced and trusted doula and our very special birthing programme, I was never in any doubt we were doing the right thing. I was frightened then angered by the words of my doctor and upset by the reaction of some friends, but I never once doubted my instincts to birth Danuta at home using hypnosis. I can't wait to give her a brother or sister."

George Longland, UK

In my experience, there is only one motivation, and that is desire. No reasons or principle contain it or stand against it – Jane Smiley

Step 3 – Know you can do it – trust your instincts

The third step is all about getting back to basics – rekindling and building the trust that your body was designed for this and that your body really does know how to birth your baby. It is about getting back to your instincts and moving on from wanting to "control" the birth, to handing it back to your primal mind and body.

Sadly, in our society, we have stopped using our instincts the way we used to and often rely on external factors to quash the messages our bodies are telling us. For many people, as soon as they have a headache they take a pill rather than think about what might be causing the headache and what they can do to change the cause, for example drinking more, relaxing, eating properly, and so on. To stop getting pregnant, we take a pill to artificially control our cycle, so we are no longer connected to nature's cycles.

A mum's experience

"The contractions started on the due date, so it took a while for me to accept that they actually were contractions and not wind :o). I kept doing the breathing and counting and 'turning the dial down' to lessen the perception of pain. When the contractions came closer and closer, we called the midwifery unit (in total three times), who kept saying, 'It's too early to come' – basically, I was too calm and controlled when they talked to me. Eventually, I had had it and said to my husband that it was time to call our baby's godfather so that he could drive us to the hospital.

I'm glad we listened to my instincts rather than the professionals. At the examination I was 8 cm dilated and the midwife who had told me to stay at home only had the expression of 'Whoops!' on her face. A little after that we met our lovely boy. Thank you!! Brilliant help."

Maggie Darwin, UK

Youth fades; love droops; the leaves of friendship fall; a mother's secret hope outlives them all – Oliver Wendell Holmes

Even when they get pregnant, many women are aware of changes in their body, but do not actually believe they are pregnant until they wee on a stick and see the small blue line, and some even do not believe they really have a baby in their tummy until they see it on an ultrasound screen.

So what does instinct mean?

The *Collins Dictionary* definition of instinct is "inborn intuitive power"; in her book *Instinctive Birth*, Val Clarke says:

> Instinct lies within you and you may experience it as a physical, emotional or psychological feeling ... Instinct is very strong and powerful. It is deeply embedded in the mind and is active from a time before birth. Most of our primal instincts are written in our genes and form a part of human survival.[1]

Naturally, many women do become more in tune with their bodies during their pregnancy, for example going off certain foods that their body does not like, taking more time to rest, drinking more water, and so on. However, that is different from being in tune with your instincts, which tend to be more emotional or mental.

On some levels we respond instinctively many times a day; for example, if a car brakes in front of you, you get an instant adrenalin rush which influences your actions. There is no conscious input – it is purely instinct and is managed by your subconscious. When you are pregnant, you instinctively want to protect your baby by placing a hand on your stomach, or rubbing you tummy.

During the journey of motherhood, you will rely on your instincts as a woman more now than at any other time. You are hard-wired to assume the role of the nurturing, protective mother. And yet many women feel that they cannot get in tune with their instincts – it is as if too much intellect and too much activity in the neocortex has somehow blocked their ability to trust their instincts. For several generations, women have come to rely on the "system" to tell them what they should be feeling, what is right and wrong, how many times their baby should move, what position their baby should be in, where they should give birth, and so on. It is no wonder that women

> ### Did you know?
> In the 1600's, doctors told husbands to fulfil their wives' cravings and desires, as, if they were not met, it would lead to miscarriage.

Train your head and hands to do, your head and heart to dare
– Joseph Seamon Cotter, Jr.

A mum's experience

"My first birth had been long and traumatic. I had tokophobia (phobia of pregnancy and birth) which was pretty much under control, until I had drugs (gas and air and pethidine) and then an argument with the midwives during second stage (they hadn't read my birth plan and didn't take my phobia seriously). This escalated into a panic attack and jeopardised the birth. Fortunately, Sam was born five hours later, safe and well. However, this left me very traumatised and concerned about getting pregnant and facing a second birth.

When I was pregnant the second time, I listened to the Pregnancy Relaxation one during the first half of pregnancy – this was a great bit of 'me' time and so relaxing (I often fell asleep), and I sailed through the first twenty-six weeks.

But it was the Birth Preparation track that was the real miracle maker. I went from being anxious about experiencing birth again (I had already arranged an action plan with the hospital for an epidural for the delivery) to deciding that I wanted a natural home birth, and felt confident that my body could handle it.

I went on to have the most amazing, relaxed water birth at home, with my husband by my side. At times it was tough, but mostly I felt relaxed and focused on what needed to be done, and happy just to follow my instincts.

Ian and I had talked through the aspects of the Natal Hypnotherapy techniques that I felt would work best for me, and worked out a script accordingly ('3, 2, 1, relax, Fran' was fantastic) and it made the birth a joint effort. It was quite a speedy birth. I was 1 cm dilated at 7 a.m. and Jack was born at 10.14 a.m. – a healthy and calm little boy.

The last six months have been a joy. Not only has it been wonderful to bond with him after such a fantastic birth experience, it has helped me to come to terms with my first birth – a burden has finally been lifted.

I would recommend these techniques wholeheartedly to anyone (and regularly do!). I actually cannot convey in words how much this positive birth experience has changed my life, and I will always be grateful to you for your advice and your tools."

Fran Benson, UK

Two roads diverged in a wood, and I took the one less travelled by, and that has made all the difference – Robert Frost

sometimes feel overpowered by "the system" and lack confidence in their own instincts.

However, those instincts are still within you. As Dr. Christiane Northrup says:

> Awaken that still, small, intuitive voice in all of us, that voice of our own body that we have been forced to ignore through our culture's illness, misinformation and dysfunction.[2]

By regaining the trust in your instincts, it will help you feel more in tune with your body and more in tune with your baby. This will help you learn to trust that your body really does know what it is doing, that it knows how to grow a beautiful baby, that it knows how to produce all the right hormones to trigger off the birth and that it will wait until your baby is ready to be born.

We have been so clouded by the belief that the medical world knows our bodies better than ourselves, and yet, as Northrup says:

> When we realign with our inner guidance and stop judging our bodies and our feelings as bad when they are offering us information, we are on the pathway to a life filled with growth and delight.[3]

Remember that our bodies, the way we grow, develop and birth our babies, and our babies' needs have not changed at all in millenia. What has changed is our levels of intellect, reasoning and analysis – all of which can easily overpower our natural instincts.

How many times have you had an instinctive thought about something, only to ignore it and then later regret not taking action on your initial thought?

How to do it – "What would Mrs. Stone Age have done?"

When you are faced with a decision or something you are unsure about, stop for a moment, close your eyes (if it is safe to do so!), tune into the feeling you are having or the sound of your heart beating, and ask yourself the question – what should I do? What feels right? Why do I have this problem?

Give yourself a moment to allow any instinctive response to come to the surface. **Always** take the first thing that pops up. Often we dismiss that and allow our conscious thinking brain

There are no speed limits on the road to excellence – David Johnson

to take over with a "yes, but ...". Make a note of what the first feeling or thought was. Even if you chose to do something else, that is OK – you have connected with your instinctive response.

Throughout all my pregnancies and my parenting journey, whenever I have been faced with a decision or concern, my first question to myself has always been:

"What would Mr. and Mrs. Stone Age have done?"

Would they have tried to force their baby to be born before it was ready?
Would they have cut the cord straight away?
Would they have put their babies in a cot?
Would they have kept their babies at a distance from them for long periods of time?
Would they have given up breastfeeding before their baby could eat?
Would they have given them food before they had teeth?

Quite often that would give me the answer I was looking for.

Using hypnosis to increase your trust and be more instinctive

One of the most effective ways of becoming more in tune with your instincts is through the use of hypnosis. By regularly communicating with your subconscious, you will learn to listen to your body, to trust your body, to tune in to the millions of years of birthing knowledge in your DNA, and so ultimately reduce fear and allow yourself to birth instinctively.

When you begin to practise hypnosis, you are not only becoming more instinctive and reducing any fears, you will also begin to get an increased sense of empowerment that you are in control of how you prepare for birth, and that this is something you are doing yourself, which will help create the change that you want.

During pregnancy and birth, many women often feel as if they are on a conveyor belt, a small part in a big system – seeing different midwives, hearing all kinds of dos and don'ts, reading all kinds of horror stories and traumas associated with pregnancy and birth, and so on. As your pregnancy progresses, the harder it becomes to let all that simply "bounce" off you and to allow yourself to trust your body simply to get on with the wonderful job of growing and developing your beautiful baby.

However, when women begin practising hypnosis, so much of the associated anxiety becomes less pronounced, all the advice and all the horror stories seem more distanced, and

We may run, walk, stumble, drive, or fly, but let us never lose sight of the reason for the journey, or miss a chance to see a rainbow on the way – Gloria Gaither

women comment on how calm, centred and at peace they feel — especially the women who were particularly anxious before. It is as if the ancient, primal part of your brain is enabling your need to trust and stay calm, thus blocking out the neocortical activity which is full of all the "what ifs" and things that could go wrong.

You soon begin to understand that all that worry and concern does not actually change anything – they are all just thoughts, which, if anything, can be damaging to you and your baby's mental and emotional well-being.

Did you know?

In 1705 in England, women were encouraged to have a healthy pregnancy by moderating their diets, sleeping as much as possible and not wearing corsets. Drinks made up of cinnamon, nutmeg, sugar and eggs were served to warm and strengthen the mother-to-be.

So if there is nothing that you can do about it right now, then there is absolutely no benefit in worrying about it.

In the very rare instances when there is something to be concerned about, those mothers that are in tune with their instincts simply "know". Many women have presented themselves to the hospital or to the midwives, saying that there is something that needs attention, and they are usually right.

How can you learn to do hypnosis yourself?

There are several avenues you can choose if you wish to learn and practise hypnosis for birth.

1. Attend a course with a qualified Natal Hypnotherapy practitioner.

Attending a course will give you hands-on experience, guidance and support from a qualified practitioner; additional tools and techniques to help you and your birth partner during the birth; the opportunity to ask questions and formulate your own plan, and to create your own bespoke scripts, affirmations and suggestions, which are tailored to you and your birth partner; and the chance to meet like-minded couples and to have a support network, including your practitioner and the other couples on your course (see appendix for more details).

The significant problems we face cannot be resolved at the same level of thinking we were at when we created them – Albert Einstein

2. Use a self-hypnosis track

As with any skill, the more you practise, the better you get. Everyone who wants to benefit from hypnosis for birth should regularly practise self-hypnosis, and a pre-prepared track is a safe, easy and wonderfully relaxing way to do this. The Natal Hypnotherapy range has been tailored to cover most types of birth including home births, vaginal births after a Caesarean, twins' births and even preparing for a Caesarean birth.

They can be listened to in your own time, in your own home and of course during the birth itself. One of the many bonuses of practising hypnosis throughout your pregnancy is that you take time out to actually slow down, relax and spend time focusing on your baby.

Many women have commented that the tracks are a great "excuse" or reason to take time out to relax, which they may not otherwise have done (see appendix for more details).

3. Visit a qualified Hypnotherapist.

If you have any very specific concerns, fears or trauma from previous experiences, you may wish to see a qualified hypnotherapist for a one-to-one session. To find an appropriate therapist, call a few in your area and have a chat or a free consultation first. The most important thing is that you feel confident and trusting of the therapist. It is of course particularly useful if the hypnotherapist has had experience of working with birth-related hypnosis. The majority of women would not need to see a hypnotherapist for more than four sessions. Be wary of anyone who says you will need more than that to achieve a positive outcome.

4. Write your own birth hypnosis script.

There are many benefits to writing your own script, as it enables you to tailor it to your exact needs, concerns and plans for the birth. Using your own name and the names of your partner, midwife, doula or even your baby can be particularly powerful.

Tip: You can use the following guidelines to write a script for anything – remembering people's names, becoming a non-smoker, getting better sleep or creating any change.

The important thing is this: to be able at any moment to sacrifice what we are for what we could become – Charles DuBois

Writing your own birth hypnosis script

1. Think of your outcome	2. Make a mind map	3. Write out your script	4. Review and improve	5. Record and upload

If you wish to write your own hypnosis programme, there are a few important pointers to remember:

1. Think of your outcome – Ask for what you want and not what you don't want

> *'Would you tell me, please, which way I ought to go from here?'*
> *'That depends a good deal on where you want to get to,'* said the cat.
> *'I don't care much where …'* said Alice.
> *'Then it doesn't matter which way you go,'* said the cat.
>
> *Alice in Wonderland*, Lewis Carroll

Always state your goals or your outcome in the positive. Remember the mind cannot NOT do something – it will always see the action first and then you consciously negate it.

For example: whatever you do, do not think of a pink elephant. What happened? The brain will first see the pink elephant and then you will try to cancel it out. Or another example: the cat is not chasing the dog. Again, the brain cannot not do something.

Therefore, the more you can focus on what you DO want, the more your mind will have a positive focus. In addition, if you know what you want and where you are heading, your subconscious mind has an outcome or focus to move towards, and so reacts more accurately, as it has a path to follow.

For your birthing script, focus on the actual **outcome** rather than the process, location, type of birth, etc. Not all of those are something you can 'control', so your overall outcome may be "a calm birth", "a peaceful birth", or a "calm birth, calm baby".

The most wasted of all days is one without laughter – E. E. Cummings

2. Creating a mind map

Creating a mind map is a great way to put down all your thoughts and hopes for the birth. It's not a "birth plan" – it is not to be used as a wish-list of what you do and do not want.

It is an excellent way for you to consolidate all that you have learnt using this book or on the Natal Hypnotherapy course and to focus on how you would like to be responding, feeling, thinking, and acting during the birth.

Once you have set your outcome, write this in the centre of a mind map. Then go through each phase of the birth and think about how you would like to be feeling or responding, what kind of activities you may be doing, and how you may be reacting to what is happening.

With a mind map, don't worry about sentences, grammar, repetition, etc – just use it as a time to 'brain dump' all of your thoughts. Use colours, pictures, arrows – be creative and have fun with it. You may find you use lots of the same words, such as relax; feel calm; smile; 3, 2, 1, relax …; more and more; etc.

Once you have filled in all the sections, leave it for a few days before you start writing it out in full. You may wish to add to it, brighten it up or make it more creative. Some people like to put theirs up at home – maybe in the bedroom or on the back of the bathroom door – as a constant reminder of all the wonderful positive thoughts and feelings.

3. Writing your script

Once you have filled in your mind map and feel happy that you have thought through all the things you would like to be feeling and the ways you would like to respond, it is time to write out your suggestions in full. When this is done, you or your birth partner can record it onto a CD or MP3; then, you only need to lie back, listen and relax.

When creating your own programme, these are the basic steps to include:

Relaxation and breathing (see step 2)
- Take yourself to a deeply relaxed state.
- Relax all the muscles within your body.
- Focus on your breathing – breathing down to your abdomen quietly and rhythmically.
- Allow your mind to focus on your body.

The probability that we may fail in the struggle ought not to deter us from the support of a cause that we believe is just – Abraham Lincoln

An example of a birth-related mind map

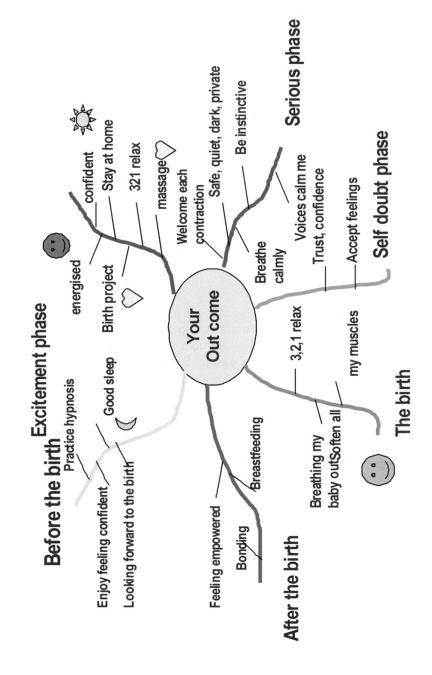

Special place or visualisation (see chapter 8)

- Use or create somewhere really special to you.
- Safe, peaceful, calm.
- Pay attention to the detail around you.
- Make it vivid and real.

Your birth (re-read chapter 2)

- Imagine seeing and experiencing yourself going through the physical process of giving birth step by step.
- Make it as detailed as possible.
- Lots of post-hypnotic triggers.
- Use your name, your partner's name, your midwife's name (if you know her).
- Use things specific to you, such as the name you have given your child or your home surroundings.
- Take your story right through to holding your baby in your arms, releasing the placenta and enjoying the amazing feeling of becoming a mother.

Exit

This is done by simply counting slowly from 1 to 5, with the following suggestions for each number:

1. Restore sensations to their true perspective. You have full co-ordination, flexibility and control from the top of your head to the tips of your toes.
2. Restore all sounds to their true perspective.
3. Place yourself back in the room, being aware of what is to your left and right, above and below.
4. Bring with you and keep all the benefits of this experience.
5. Eyes open and wide awake.

A mother understands what a child does not say – Jewish proverb

How to write a good script

What you are going to do is write a "story" of your forthcoming birth from a very physiological and emotional aspect. It is not about what will be going on around you or where you are, but more about what will be happening inside your body and how you would like to respond to it. By going through this, it is a bit like going through a dress rehearsal in your mind, so that you can practise over and over again how you would like to respond when you go into labour for real.

This is a technique used a great deal by athletes or top performers. They will see themselves at a time in the future on the day of a big race or a major presentation. They will run through their steps leading up to the moment, focusing on how they want to be responding and feeling. They will then see, feel, and experience themselves going through the event, imagining what they will be saying, how they will be moving, what they will be thinking. They will ultimately see and feel themselves being successful – crossing the finishing line, hearing the applause.

Visualization is another tool that Olympic athletes use to get their minds in shape for competition. In this technique, athletes mentally rehearse exactly what they have to do to win. Sports psychologists say that visualization boosts athletes' confidence by forcing them to picture themselves winning. It also helps them concentrate on their physical moves, rather than on distractions around them.[4]

When writing your programme, keep the following in mind:

Choose your words carefully

Choosing the right words is extremely important. Remember that the subconscious takes words very literally and is particularly open to positive suggestions. It is therefore important to use words which have a positive feel.

So, to get the best response from your mind, use positive, progressive language to get the desired outcome. Remember that suggestions work best when you have intense emotion combined with relaxation.

What words will make you feel good? It is often useful to make a list of the words that appeal to you. You can use a thesaurus to help. Ask yourself, "How would I like to feel?"

> *To us, family means putting your arms around each other and being there*
> *– Barbara Bush*

Here are some words you may like to use in your suggestions:

Exciting	Powerful	Serene	Good
Calm	Fantastic	Amazing	Peace
Relaxed	Instinctive	Harmony	Balance
Healthy	Confident	Vibrant	Wonderful
Happy	Trusting	Assured	Joyful

When writing suggestions, avoid using the following words:

Words that illicit bad feeling
Words that are ambiguous
Words that are limiting, restrictive or disempowering

Can't	Want	Won't	Should
Must	Try	Ought to	Don't
Have to	Pain	Fear	Must not

Always write what you want, and not what you do not want; for example, instead of saying, "I do not want to feel any pain," you could say, "I feel calm, relaxed and able to manage all the sensations."

Visualisations

Your hypnosis programme will be made stronger and more powerful by adding plenty of vivid, emotive visualisations. These could include:

Your special place (see chapter 8) – including a "special place" is a very powerful technique, as it is a way of training your mind to literally switch off from your daily life and go off to a dreamy state very quickly.

Your internal body – You should include imagery of exactly what is happening inside your body during the birthing. For example, seeing, feeling or experiencing the long muscles of the uterus reaching down to gently pull open the round muscles of the cervix; imagining that all the contractions are massaging the baby; the baby pressing down and opening the cervix.

In time of test, family is best – Burmese proverb

Metaphor – Many women like to include metaphors for contractions, such as experiencing yourself riding above your contractions, like riding on the crest of a wave or being a seagull above a stormy sea, soaring over the waves, but very much in touch with, aware of and in view of them. Think of something that has power and beauty and a natural force. Other metaphors women like are for the opening of the cervix: a very common one is of a flower opening slowly, petal by petal.

Visual triggers

At some points in the birthing, you may want to focus your attention externally. You may wish to include suggestions about looking at your partner's face, a picture on the wall, a reminder of your soon-to-be-born baby (perhaps a toy), an object in the room, or even a crack in the plaster. Turn this into a post-hypnotic suggestion (see below), for example, "every time I look into my partner's face it gives me the confidence I need to trust my body even more"; "seeing the picture on the wall encourages me to relax even more deeply".

Auditory triggers

Sounds such as music, the soothing voice of the birth partner, humming or other sounds also act as good triggers for deep relaxation. For example: "with every note of the music I feel even more at ease"; "the sound of my partner's voice is so encouraging and loving and reminds me of the wonderful life we will have with our baby".

Remember, you can also write suggestions to counteract any negative noises; for example, if there are sounds outside the room that are not helpful, use the following suggestion: "for any sounds which are not useful to you, you become less and less aware of them, as they only serve to help you become more and more relaxed and focus on the amazing process of birth taking place within your body".

Olfactory triggers

If you like the smell of aromatherapy oils, then use them as a trigger for relaxation. For example, one of the suggestions may be: "the warm, comforting smell of lavender helps all my muscles to stay soft and relaxed, allowing my uterus to work effectively and efficiently to allow my baby to be born". A great tip is to burn the oils you plan on using during the birth whilst listening to or practising your hypnosis.

Kinaesthetic triggers

During the labour, you may love to be touched or may want to be left completely alone. However, it is useful to build in some suggestions based on feelings or touch, for example, "every time I feel the gentle touch of my partner, my muscles respond, relaxing, softening and letting go of all tension"; "the warm feeling of the hot-water bottle takes me off to the beautiful sun-drenched beach".

We all grow up with the weight of history on us. Our ancestors dwell in the attics of our brains as they do in the spiraling chains of knowledge hidden in every cell of our bodies – Shirley Abbott

Post-hypnotic suggestions (see chapter 7)

Include as many post-hypnotic suggestions as possible, that is, 'when xxx happens, you react with yyy'. The xxx are things that you know for a fact will happen, e.g. having contractions, feelings getting more intense, your body opening, your baby moving down, and so on. And the yyy is how you respond to each of those occurrences, e.g. staying calm and relaxed, breathing deeply, trusting your body, and so on.

This is a good time to revisit your hopes and fears and to address any particular fears.

So, for example, if you have a fear of injections, you can give your subconscious a new response; instead of tensing, you can give yourself the following suggestions:

> *"When you see the needle, your whole body softens and relaxes as you allow all your muscles to become wonderfully soft. You trust that there is a good reason for needing this injection so that ultimately both you and your baby will benefit. The feeling of the needle on your skin is cool and precise and naturally you take a deep breath, saying the words, '3, 2, 1, relax'. You are aware of the sensation and yet are surprised that you can accept it and acknowledge that it will only be for a few short seconds."*

As you go through each phase of the birth, use the knowledge you have of what is happening to your body (see chapter 2) combined with your instincts as to how you would like to feel at each stage. Think about what will be happening to you, your body and your baby. The way you handle the birth will be far more important than the environment and circumstances in which you birth your baby.

Here are some examples of suggestions you can use:

> *"With the very first contraction, you feel so calm and yet wonderfully excited as you know that soon you will be meeting your baby."*

> *"As the sensations become more regular, you accept each one as taking you one step closer to meeting your baby."*

> *"With each sensation your mind becomes creative at taking you off to a special place in which you feel wonderfully calm and at ease."*

> *"As the sensations become more intense, your breathing becomes more focused as you relax your body even more."*

A new baby is like the beginning of all things – wonder, hope, a dream of possibilities
– Eda J. Le Shan

"You might be surprised that each sensation seems and feels shorter and shorter and easier and more comfortable. The time between sensations feels long enough for you to have all the rest you need, so you can feel delightfully refreshed and energised when the next sensation begins."

"And you might be surprised that no matter how fast or slow the sensations come, you always feel on top of them, riding the waves, as you know that each one lasts such a short time and will always come to an end."

Think about anything or any occurrence which might lead to an increase of anxiety or an increase of adrenalin – e.g., the journey to the hospital, meeting new people, having an internal examination – and then think about how you could turn it around to use that situation to have a positive outcome.

"On the journey to the hospital, the sights and sounds help you stay calm, focused and relaxed. Each time the car stops or turns, your body instantly relaxes even more and you breathe deep down to where your baby lies."

"Every new face you meet reminds you of the confidence you have in your body to birth your baby."

And, of course, make sure you use lots and lots of triggers and responses, such as:

"Every time you hear the words '3, 2, 1, relax', you sink into an even deeper state of calm."

"Each time you feel the special touch of your partner, your shoulders drop and you breathe down to your baby."

"The wonderful smell of lavender makes you feel so at ease and happy that your body knows exactly what it is doing!"

As your subconscious is very connected to your name, it is useful to use your name in the suggestions.

Having a baby changes the way you view your in-laws. I love it when they come to visit now. They can hold the baby and I can go out – Matthew Broderick

Additional pain management with the comfort dial

There are several pain-management techniques you can add to your programme that are similar to those used by dentists who perform dental surgery with no anaesthetic.

The following is the comfort dial, which many women have found invaluable during the birth.

> *You imagine a dial with numbers 1 to 10. As the sensations increase, the meter reading goes up … However, you now have the ability within you to turn back the dial to a number and feeling that is comfortable for you … As the dial goes down, a numbing sensation takes the place of the pressure … leaving the area numb and comfortable … numb and comfortable … You can even turn the dial to 1, so you only register the slightest sensation … still aware of what is happening, but maintaining the sensations at a comfortable level.*

Remember to take your story right the way through to holding your baby in your arms and releasing the placenta.

4. Review and improve

Once you have written out your suggestions in full, put on your editing hat.

Have any words entered without your intention?

Are you happy with the finished result?

How does it make you feel when you read it?

Are there any parts which do not make you feel confident?

Do not proceed if there is any doubt about your suggestions. When in doubt, think about your suggestion and then either take it out or rewrite it. Do what you can to remove negativity or ambiguity, and only then proceed.

Children seldom misquote you. They more often repeat word for word what you should not have said – Mea Maloo

5. Uploading your programme

Once you are happy with your script, it is time to begin using it. The easiest way is to record the script so that you can then simply lie back and listen. It is a good idea to ask your birth partner to record it for you, so that you associate the triggers and relaxation with your partner's voice. Also, it is always beneficial to have calm, relaxing music in the background, so that, again, you associate that particular music with a sense of calm and relaxation.

Here are some tips for the person recording the session:

1. Begin in your usual speaking voice and then allow your voice to become quieter, softer and more relaxed, so that you are speaking more slowly. It may seem unnatural in the beginning, but aim to go more slowly than you think you should.
2. Add pauses and gaps between the words and sentences.
3. Lengthen the words, adding emphasis on key words such as "relax".
4. Make your voice quite monotone.

I then recommend that you listen to it as often as possible, leading up to once a day for the last few weeks of pregnancy.

Even if you do not go on to record and use your script, the process of creating your own script is a wonderful way to prepare for the birth, as you are consciously as well as subconsciously making the shift towards increasing your trust and confidence in your ability to give birth.

If you do not feel confident in your ability to write a script, you can attend a course or speak to your local practitioner for support and guidance. In addition, there is the full range of Natal Hypnotherapy tracks that you can use. These include birth preparation ones for home births, for hospital/birth centres, for twins, for vaginal births after a Caesarean, and for those preparing for a Caesarean (see appendix for more details).

---

[1] Clarke, V., *Instinctive Birth*, Carroll & Brown Publishers Limited (25 March 2005).

[2] Christiane Northrup, 2002, *Women's Bodies, Women's Wisdom*, Bantem Dell.

[3] Christiane Northrup, 2002, *Women's Bodies, Women's Wisdom*, Bantem Dell.

[4] Fiona McCormack, "Mind Games", *Scholastic Scope*, Vol. 54, Iss. 10, New York: 23 Jan 2006.

I know how to do anything – I'm a mom – Roseanne Barr

A mum's experience

"My son Hector was born on 2 April. Things started off quite slowly, as my body seemed to be warming up for labour. For that whole time of early labour, I was completely relaxed, and I kept on getting up to walk during each contraction. Once my contractions were really regular and coming every five minutes, I called the Birth Centre at the hospital to ask if I should come in. The midwife said that I sounded too calm and was probably not very advanced. She advised me to lie down and rest for when the real 'active' labour started.

I did as I was told, but the contractions kept on coming, and at one point I looked at my husband and was almost in tears, not so much because of the labour, but because of the indecision about when to go into hospital! When I stood up to use the toilet at 7 p.m., my water broke, and we then decided that we had to go in. When I arrived at the hospital I was in full-force labour, and after about an hour and a half of really tough contractions (this was really the hardest part of the labour), I suddenly had this overwhelming desire to push.

The midwife didn't seem to believe me, but when she examined me, to her astonishment she said that I was almost there. I asked if I could get into the birth pool when I started pushing. I tried to use gas and air a couple of times, but soon realised that I didn't need it. My baby was born at 10.45 p.m. underwater in the birth pool. I had had such a good birth experience; my incredibly beautiful baby was there – in my arms – and I was meeting him on the outside for the first time.

I believe that my positive birth experience was due to the Natal Hypnotherapy and Active Birth yoga that I did in preparation. From about week 36 of my pregnancy I listened to the preparation-for-birth hypnotherapy CD daily, and actually the first time that I listened to it, I was brought to tears because I was so moved by its message! I believe that these positive messages about giving birth gave me confidence in my body and in the incredible force of nature that dictates exactly what to do in the moment while going through such an intense experience – that is, if we trust and listen.

My son was extremely calm the entire time, and he didn't even cry when he first came out of the water. Now, at three months, he is still a very calm baby, perhaps

Any mother could perform the jobs of several air-traffic controllers with ease
– Lisa Alther

partly because of having such a calm birth, and partly because of the positive messages that he received through the hypnotherapy while in utero. I feel that such a smooth birth experience was a beautiful gift to give to him and to my husband.

And it was an even more incredible gift for me to be able to completely trust in my body to do it. Following my instinct pulled me through, and I look back on it and see a golden light surrounding my son's birth story. I have now joined the countless women who have come before me on this journey, and I look back on it with pride – not so much pride in myself, but in the incredible perfection that is my body. A mother's body is another manifestation of Mother Nature herself."

Jessica Sequera, UK

Step 4 – Acquire practical skills

In addition to using and practising hypnosis, there are many practical exercises and ways to prepare for a comfortable birth. It is important to remember that all women respond differently to birthing depending on their bodies, their environment, their sense of readiness, their coping styles, and their goals and expectations.

It is therefore useful to gather and prepare as many different coping strategies and practical ways to help yourself during the birth as possible. That way, there are bound to be a few specific tools that will work well for you on the day.

As you prepare and mentally rehearse for the birth, learning various comfort measures and then adapting them to suit you will be of great help during the birth itself.

So, first of all, think about all the different ways that you like to relax.

What do you enjoy doing?

How do you know you are relaxed?

What things make you feel calm and at ease?

In what environments do you feel most happy?

Is it certain kinds of music, or a massage, soothing voices, aromatherapy smells, a bath or shower, meditation, prayer, chanting, a walk on a beach, or a swing in a hammock?

Did you know?

Make a list of those things and include them in your mind map and hypnosis programme. In addition, you can use any of the following techniques without ever having done any hypnosis at all.

Music is played throughout labour for the Navajo women of the American south west.

Children are our most valuable natural resource – Herbert Hoover

Comfort measures during birth

Your needs and emotional state are going to vary a great deal throughout the birth, so it is useful to look at a wide range of comfort measures with your birth partner, so that, between you, you have a "tool kit" that you can dip into at different times.

Many women successfully employ both tuning-in and distraction techniques. For instance, in early labour you may wish to relax, breathe slowly, rhythmically and easily through your contractions, close your eyes, and visualise either something very soothing and pleasant or the uterine contractions opening the cervix and pressing the baby downward.

As the birthing becomes more intense, you may continue in this way or you may simply focus on your breathing while counting slowly to ten. Then, during self-doubt, when contractions are very intense and close, you may find you need to change your coping strategy to be more external. You may want to open eyes, focus outside (perhaps on your partner's face, a photograph, or even a mark on the wall), and follow external directions, such as your partner guiding your breathing with verbal directions, with hand signals, or by breathing with you.

Using your mind, thoughts and attention

During contractions, it is wonderfully beneficial to focus your attention on something specific. By activating different parts of your brain, you are intercepting the nerve impulses from your uterus to your brain, thereby reducing the intensity of the contractions. You have probably already experienced this many times, for example when you have had a headache and then have watched a good film and suddenly noticed that it has gone, or, if you are a sports person with an injury, when you have been on the field and have realised that you do not notice the pain at all.

The many visualisations and suggestions in your hypnosis programme will help you to do this automatically. However, even if you have not practised hypnosis, it is useful to go through these with your partner, so that they can reiterate or suggest them to you during the birth. Use the pages at the end of the book to write down the key ones as a prompt for your birth partner.

People often say that motivation doesn't last. Well, neither does bathing – that's why we recommend it daily – Zig Ziglar

Tip: You can even transfer these onto small cards, so that your partner has a pack of cards with all the "tools and techniques" written down.

Your special place
Go to the special place you have practised during your pregnancy. This might be the same or it might be different.

Your internal body
You might visualise exactly what is happening inside your body – the long muscles of the uterus reaching down to gently pull open the round muscles of the cervix, the contractions massaging the baby, and the baby pressing down and opening the cervix.

A mum's experience

"During the birth of my first son, my main memory is of travelling all over the world, going to marvellous places, and reliving experiences. We had chosen to have our baby at home and had prepared the small barn next to the house as the birthing room. It was in the middle of winter, but it was so warm and cosy, with a big wood-burning stove in one corner and a huge cast-iron bath constantly filled up with hot water.

When I was in the 'serious' part of the labour, my husband Clint was absolutely fantastic and came up with the idea of reminding me of all the places we had travelled together. At the beginning of each contraction, he would simply say the word of a town or region we had been to, and in my mind I was able to go straight there and remember everything I could about it – the sounds, the smells, the scenery, people we met, and so on – which completely took my mind off the contractions. He carried on doing this for what seemed like hours, and soon I was actually looking forward to each contraction, wondering where in the world I would go next!

Even the midwives said that they were also looking forward to each one, as it felt like an adventure for them, too!"

Sophie Mazzotti, South Africa

A mother is a person who, seeing there are only four pieces of pie for five people, promptly announces she never did care for pie – Tenneva Jordan

Metaphor

Many women like to imagine a different scenario that matches the emotions and feelings of contractions, such as experiencing yourself riding above your contractions, as if you are riding on the crest of a wave or are a gull above a stormy sea, soaring over, but still very much in touch with, the contractions.

External focal point

At some points in the birthing, you may want to focus your attention externally. You may wish to look at your partner's face, a picture on the wall, a reminder of the baby (perhaps a toy), an object in the room, or even a crack in the plaster. Some women focus on the same thing for many contractions; others change focal points often.

A great way of staying in the moment and yet knowing that each contraction only lasts a short time is to focus on a line, such as the edge of a window or lines on a floor board, and then to follow that line, slowly starting at one end and finishing at the other by the time the contraction finishes.

Auditory stimulus

Focusing on sounds such as music, the soothing voice of your birth partner, a tape recording of various environmental sounds (surf, rain, a babbling brook), repeating rhythms, or other sounds.

Many women naturally use sounds to help them through contractions. When a woman opens her throat, vocalises, hums, moans, or groans through a contraction, she is also opening her birth canal. It can be a really powerful way of releasing tension and relaxing the body.

Mental activity

Many women naturally choose some repetitive mental activity which focuses their thoughts. Counting is a very popular choice, for example counting each breath, counting up to ten and then back down again, counting the seconds of each contraction. Others choose repetitive actions, such as repeating a song, a poem or a chant.

In the weeks leading up to the birth, take time to practise going through the breathing with a stimulus exercise (see step 2). As you and your partner practise breathing and relaxing together through the contractions, use the different attention-focusing techniques described above. You will probably discover a preference for some over others. Be ready to explore more than one if a particular focus loses its appeal during the birth.

The greatest part of our happiness depends on our dispositions, not our circumstances – Martha Washington

Physical comfort measures

Movement

Research and instinct have shown that the worst position for both the mother and the baby during labour is for the mother to be lying flat on her back. This is not only uncomfortable, but can cause more difficulties and can slow down labour. The reason for this is that the largest blood vessel in your body runs up and down your back, behind the uterus. If you think of the weight of your baby and your uterus as being the equivalent to a heavy bowling ball, you can easily imagine what happens to the large blood vessel when you lie on your back. There is undue pressure as it is pinched between the pelvic bones and your back.

As a result, the circulation is interfered with and so is the supply of oxygen and nutrients to your baby. This compression may, over time, reduce the blood flow to the placenta, resulting in the baby getting less oxygen. When a baby is short of oxygen, there is a risk of what is known as a 'foetal distress' developing – a common reason for a Caesarean section or the use of forceps or ventouse to deliver the baby quickly.

During early labour, the contractions will be more effective and more comfortable if you keep upright and move around. This is because the uterus naturally tilts forward during a contraction. When you are upright and leaning forward, you help the uterus to do its work without resistance. In addition, there is a much better blood supply to the placenta when you are upright, compared to lying down.

Being upright allows the bones and ligaments of the pelvis to move and adjust to ease the passage for the baby. This is especially true of the coccyx or tailbone, as it can move backwards during the last stages of labour, thus increasing the amount of space for the baby to move through the birth canal. This cannot happen if a woman is lying on her back.

So, moving around during your birth is an extremely useful comfort measure. Changing your position – sitting, kneeling, standing, lying down, getting on your hands and knees, and walking – all help relieve discomfort and facilitate the birth by adding the benefits of gravity and changes in the shape of the pelvis. Swaying from side to side, rocking, or other rhythmic movements are both comforting and a great way to get the baby into a good position.

If you think you're too small to have an impact, try going to bed with a mosquito
– Anita Roddick

Partner: As labour progresses, she may be wrapped up in herself and will be inclined to stay in one position. If she is relaxed and all is progressing well, then it is fine for her to stay as she is. However, if you see any signs of an adrenalin blip, remind her gently to move onto her side or to sit up, move around a little and use the birthing ball.

Massage and Touch

The benefits of massage have been felt by most people and have been studied by many. Massage does not just feel good. Research shows it reduces the heart rate, lowers blood pressure, increases blood circulation and lymph flow, relaxes muscles, improves range of motion, and increases endorphins, the body's natural painkillers[1].

Did you know?

In the Yucatan, massage is a regular part of women's antenatal care. This helps the woman relax and helps move the baby into the best possible position – even breech babies are turned using abdominal massage.

During massage, large amounts of these endorphins are released into the bloodstream. This explains the feeling you may have afterwards of being slightly groggy and lightheaded, but with a calm sense of well-being.

Famed Victorian physician Dr. Dowse remarked in 1887:

> The mind, which before massage is in a perturbed, restless, vacillating, and even despondent state, becomes calm, quiet, peaceful, and subdued after massage. In fact, the wearied and worried mind has been converted into a mind restful, placid, and refreshed.

Candice Pert, an expert on endorphins, is enthusiastic about the release of endorphins during massage.

> From my research with endorphins, I know the power of touch to stimulate and regulate our natural chemicals, the ones that are tailored to act at precisely the right times in exactly the appropriate dosages to maximize our feelings of health and well being.[2]

During labour, women may either love it or hate it. As a partner, it is important to pick up on her cues as to whether she is benefiting from it or not.

> *I discovered I always have choices and sometimes it's only a choice of attitude*
> *– Judith M. Knowlton*

A mum's experience

"I wanted you to know what an impact Natal Hypnotherapy had on me and the huge amount we both learnt from the course. I am so proud that I managed to give birth without any intervention and that I was so focused, and didn't even want gas and air. I had always hoped and visualised it like this, but to actually experience it was magical. Hard work but worth it!

The techniques we learnt from the course were invaluable, not only during the - actual birth, in helping me to relax, but also during the pregnancy – particularly in the last two tense weeks, when Grace was overdue. I felt extremely empowered (and confident) to make the decision not to be induced. Also, Brian was confident that he was doing the right things during the whole process to support me – 'shaking the apples' was great!

I definitely feel that Brian and myself managed and ran my labour. It was a wonderful experience!"

Brian and Anna Morgan, UK

Some women like an extremely light, even "tickly" stroking, which has the ability to release lots of the pain-numbing hormones, while others find a firmer touch more soothing. As you and your partner prepare for the birth, explore varying the pressure and rhythm of massage until you discover the most appealing stroke. Then practise it as part of your birth preparation.

During pregnancy, women often run their hand over their tummies in a light stroking motion, so you may find a gentle massage over the lower abdomen, following the lower curve of the uterus, a comforting and enjoyable feeling.

If you enjoy this kind of massage, make sure your partner uses cornstarch or oil to make their hands slide more easily. Keep the massage rhythmic, pacing it with the slow breathing.

Other types of massage, such as firm stroking, kneading (squeezing and releasing), or rubbing, are soothing and relaxing during both pregnancy and labour. Massage of the neck, shoulders, back, thighs, feet and hands can be very comforting. Work together in pregnancy to find out how and where massage is most helpful and how you plan to use it during the birth.

It is more important to know where you are going than to get there quickly
– Mabel Newcomber

Back pressure

Another helpful form of massage for birth is firm pressure, used particularly over the lower back or sacrum during contractions. In my experience as a doula, it is this form of pressure that most women really enjoy.

One technique is called sacral pressure and is especially helpful for easing any discomfort in the back during contractions. Your partner presses the heel of a hand on the sacral area of your lower back and simply holds it there for the duration of the contraction. During labour, you may be surprised at how much pressure you want, so make sure you give that feedback to your partner.

The exact spot for applying pressure varies from woman to woman and changes during labour, so it is difficult to know in advance which spot will be best. As long as you know the technique, you and your partner will be able to apply it during labour to wherever suits you Best.

You may need a surprising amount of pressure, which may be very tiring for your partner after a few hours. It is worth the effort, though, as the relief and comfort it brings can be immense. Your partner can take turns with another support person to allow him or her to take a rest.

Shaking the apples

This is a technique used by Ina May Gaskin (thank you Ina May!) and one which I have used as a doula a great deal.

What is the first thing you do if you have banged or hurt yourself?

Instinctively, you rub it vigorously, which often makes it feel better.

"Shaking the apples" simply involves standing behind the mother, as she leans on a chair or kneels over the ball or bed, and using both hands to vigorously rub the mother's back, hips, bottom, thighs and legs! This should be done between contractions and at times when she needs a boost or a change.

It is especially useful if she has had an adrenalin blip and needs to get back into the "zone". This may be due to her waters breaking and the next contraction being very intense, or it may be after a new person has come on the scene or after moving to another place to have her baby.

If you have knowledge, let others light their candles in it – Margaret Fuller

There are many benefits of using this technique. It helps with:

1. Releasing adrenalin.
2. Releasing lactic acid.
3. Releasing tension in the vital areas around the cervix and pelvis.
4. Increasing blood flow to the birthing area.
5. Helping the mum release tension all over.
6. Making her laugh!

Warm water

What is one of the first things you like to do after a long, hard day, or when you are feeling a bit under the weather? For many, it is taking a long, warm soak in the bath.

This, of course, is especially wonderful during labour. As soon as you enter warm water, your body instinctively relaxes, which makes the contractions more manageable.

A mum's experience

"I would like to say how grateful I am to you after followingyour method. I was very sceptical about what use they would be, as I would fall asleep regularly before the tracks had finished and thought that they couldn't surely be working. The bonus was that I was getting to sleep, which I was having difficulty with! But, as my due date approached, I was surprised to find that I was getting very excited (not terrified, as I was before using the tools).

When I arrived at hospital, I was admitted to a ward and was left by the midwife, who assumed that I was only having mild contractions (if any at all). I asked if I could be examined to see how far I was gone, to be told I was already 5 cm dilated and that they would get the water running to fill the pool for the water birth I wanted. The midwife was really surprised and said that I seemed far too laid-back, making me very pleased with myself. Once in the pool, the water was heavenly, and as I relaxed even more the labour progressed very quickly and my daughter was born in only a few hours, with me only having a few goes on the gas and air and having not sworn at my husband once!"

Caroline Slaney, UK

I think the key is for women not to set any limits – Martina Navratilova

The use of water as a method of pain relief was pioneered in the 1970's by Michel Odent and has increased in popularity in recent years, with most maternity units having water-birth facilities. For women choosing to have their babies at home, it has become even easier and more affordable to buy or rent a pool.

Research into the safety and efficacy of water births has shown that they are extremely safe and in many ways help women to have more instinctive and drug-free births[3,4].

Michel Odent writes:

> *The reason why kneeling or immersion in water during labour is so helpful is mysterious. What is clear is that water is often the way to reduce inhibition. We observe that during such immersion in warm water, semi-darkness is the best way to reach a high level of relaxation. Water may be a good way to reduce adrenergic secretion. Immersion in warm water with semi-darkness may also be a way to reach alpha brain wave rhythms.*[5]

According to Janet Balaskas in her book on water births[6], the benefits to a woman in labour are that being in water:

- Increases privacy
- Provides significant pain relief
- Reduces the need for drugs and interventions
- Encourages a woman's sense of control in labour
- Facilitates mobility and enables the woman to adopt optimal positions for an active birth
- Speeds up labour
- Promotes relaxation and conserves energy
- Helps to reduce perineal tears
- Is rated highly by mothers and midwives
- Encourages an easier birth for the mother and a gentler welcome for the baby

On another level, being immersed in water and cocooned in a small, private space may also be a subconscious symbol of comfort and of regression to a womb-like environment of safety and protection. My own theory is that, when in the pool, a mother is left alone; she has a safe space around her, which is so important to a birthing mammal – remember the baobab tree?

Whichever way you look at it, one thing is sure: when using water, the contractions become more efficient and so more manageable, making birth a more positive experience.

A perfect example of minority rule is a baby in the house – Milwaukee Journal

It is important not to get too hung-up on wanting a "water birth" – for some women, when it actually comes to birthing their babies, they actually want to get out of the water, as instinctively they want to be on dry land. See the use of water as a comfort measure, rather than as a predetermined outcome.

To make the most of using water during your birth, here are a few key points to remember:

1. Leave getting in the pool as long as you can. In some hospitals, the guidelines are that you should wait until you are 5 cm dilated; however, if you are not choosing to have vaginal exams and do not want to know how many centimetres you are, then simply hold off until you really feel like you need some additional support. The most important factor is that your contractions are regular and increasing in intensity. Women have gone from 3 cm to fully dilated in a very short amount of time, but the key was that their contractions were strong and regular.

2. Do not stay in the pool continually for more than two hours. It is a good idea to get out, have a walk around, go to the loo, and so on.

3. Keep the water at a temperature that is comfortable for you during the labour. Women often like the water to be a lower temperature than a normal bath. However, it is recommended that the water is approximately 36 to 37 degrees, especially for around the time the baby is born. If you are at home, make sure you are familiar with putting the pool up and knowing how long it takes to fill up, remembering to turn on the immersion heater.

If you do not have a birth pool, you can still benefit from taking a bath or a long, warm shower. In the shower, lean against the wall or sit on a towel-covered stool so that you can rest. Direct the spray where it helps most – maybe on your lower back or on your lower abdomen. When you are in the bath, cover your tummy with a warm, wet flannel or hand towel – it will stop your tummy from getting cold!

I have used water and birth pools for the births of all of my sons: one just for relaxation before and during labour, two that I actually gave birth in, and one when I only used it after the baby was born, when my son floated with me in the warm water for a good hour, whilst I drank lots of sweet tea and ate copious amounts of toast.

However, the enjoyment and pleasure we got out of the pool before and after the birth was immeasurable. In fact, a while ago, one of my sons asked if I was going to have another

The patience of a mother might be likened to a tube of toothpaste – it's never quite all gone – Author unknown

baby. When I asked him why he had asked, he said it was because he wanted to get the pool back! I am now pregnant with my fifth child, and the three older boys are as excited about getting the pool again as they are about getting a new baby brother or sister!

Heat and cold

Remember how, in old films, when a woman is having a baby, there are calls for lots of clean towels and hot water? The use of heat is part of ancient birth wisdom. We associate heat with comfort, relaxation and letting go – lying in the warm sun, relaxing in a warm bath, enjoying a sauna. Gentle heat encourages blood flow and relaxation of muscles, which of course is beneficial during labour.

When heat is applied to the low abdomen, back, groin, or perineum, it can be very soothing. There are lots of things you can use, such as a hot-water bottle, or hot compresses made up of washcloths or small towels soaked in hot water, wrung out, and quickly applied wherever you need them. As they cool, they should be replaced.

Conversely, applying a cold pack can also provide a great deal of relief, especially as your body is "hotting up" in the later stages of labour. A cold pack can be anything – an ice bag, a rubber glove filled with crushed ice, a bag of frozen peas, "instant" cold packs, or frozen gel packs (camper's "ice" or the cold packs used for athletic injuries). A cold flannel placed on the forehead, or a cold pack placed on the lower back for back pain during labour or on the perineum immediately after birth to reduce pain and swelling, feels wonderful. For cold packs to bring comfort, however, you must be feeling comfortably warm. If you are feeling chilled, a cold pack should not be used.

Use common sense in deciding how hot or cold the compresses should be. When in labour, you might easily tolerate compresses so hot or cold that they could damage your skin. Cover these with a towel to make sure that your skin is protected. You should not use a cold compress on the perineum for more than 10 to 15 minutes, as it will decrease the blood flow to the area and so slow down healing.

Aromatherapy oils

Another useful comfort measure in childbirth is the use of aromatherapy oils. In recent years, there has been increased interest in the efficacy of oils in terms of pain relief and the ability to keep the mother calm and relaxed[7].

A conscience is like a baby. It has to go to sleep before you can
– Author unknown

You can use oils for massage by mixing five or six drops in a little base oil, such as almond oil. Alternatively, they can be diluted with a few drops of water and used on an essential oil burner. They can also be added to a cold-water spray or a compress. If you cannot take a candle burner into hospital, then you can now buy electric oil burners that plug into a normal socket, or you can buy a terracotta ring that you put on top of an electric lightbulb.

Some of the most common and recommended oils for use during the labour are lavender, neroli, marjoram and rose. Another oil which has beneficial properties when used in labour is clary sage, which is supposed to encourage labour and stimulate contractions if things are very slow to start or have really slowed down during labour. However, it is advised to avoid clary sage during pregnancy.

You will probably find these basic aromatherapy essential oils at your local health-food shop or natural-remedy supplier. There are also many places that now sell specially blended oils for labour, which can often work out cheaper than buying whole bottles of each oil. Alternatively, you could consult a qualified practitioner for advice on which oils are beneficial.

Tip: if you like the smell of oils, then burn them at the same time you are practising your hypnosis, as you will make the subconscious connection with the oils and relaxation, which will be triggered when you smell the oils during the birth.

Beverages

Many women naturally lose their appetite when they begin active labour, so it is important to eat plenty of healthy, high-energy food in the last few weeks of pregnancy. The reason for this loss of appetite is that the digestive system uses a great deal of energy, which, during labour, is best diverted to the business of birthing. In addition, your digestive system will aim to clear itself to make more room for the baby to move down and out, which is why many women often have a runny tummy before labour and also vomit during labour. Some women do feel hungry during labour, but then find that they can only eat very small amounts.

What is important, though, is that you continue to take in liquids throughout the birthing process. Remember to bring a straw so that you can drink in any position you happen to be in. During your labour, you can drink water, tea, or juice, or suck on ice cubes made from frozen fruit juice or frozen puréed fruit, although it is better to avoid acidic drinks in case you need to be sick (which is quite common).

When I was a child, my mother said to me, 'If you become a soldier, you'll be a general. If you become a monk, you'll end up as the pope.' Instead I became a painter and wound up as Picasso – Pablo Picasso

Hourly trips to the bathroom to urinate will increase your comfort during contractions, as it takes away any pressure around the bladder and makes more room for the baby to descend down into the birth canal. If you have a very dry mouth, you can suck on ice cubes, a wet facecloth, a glucose tablet or a lollipop. You may also want to refresh your mouth and teeth with cold water, a toothbrush, or mouthwash.

The birthing ball

The use of a "birthing ball" or exercise ball has become very common during labour, with many maternity units having them on the ward as standard. However, the benefits you can get from using one start from early pregnancy and go right through to after your baby has been born and beyond. They are therefore a very worthwhile investment, and many women would not be without theirs.

Using the ball throughout pregnancy will help to keep your posture in the correct position, will help get your baby in a good position, and will build strength and flexibility in the supporting muscles in the spine and thighs. It is especially good in late pregnancy, when it can be uncomfortable to sit on hard chairs or get up and down from the sofa.

The birth ball is a simple yet amazing piece of equipment for any pregnant woman. In its most basic form, a woman can simply sit on the ball and instantly improve her posture, ease back pain and relax, as well as using it to exercise her pelvic floor muscles. Also, when one sits on a ball, the legs naturally drop to the sides, thus opening the pelvis to its widest diameter and adding optimal foetal positioning in preparation for labour.[8]

Benefits during pregnancy

- Simply by sitting and rolling with the ball encourages rhythmic movement and pelvic mobility.

- The softness and shape of the ball absorbs your weight and helps to prevent and relieve back strain.

- Kneeling forwards over the ball takes the weight off your back and is great practice for labour.

- As the ball is not flat, it is always moving slightly; therefore, by sitting on the ball, you will be using your inner thighs and pelvic floor muscles without even noticing.

My mother is my root, my foundation. She planted the seed that I base my life on, and that is the belief that the ability to achieve starts in your mind – Michael Jordan

- Natural movements with the ball help to gently tone your internal and external pelvic muscles.

- Sitting on the ball at your desk raises your hips higher than your knees. This encourages your baby to settle into an optimal position for birth.

A mum's experience

"Before learning Natal Hypnotherapy and doing antenatal yoga, I was all for a birth plan asking for all drugs going! However, by the end, I was so relaxed and confident I even considered a home birth with no pain relief.

My waters broke a week early, when I was having a rest in the afternoon. I was so calm, quietly breathing away on my birth ball, that my husband told my mum and the midwife that he thought the pain was OK! After an hour or so, I asked for my mum again. When she came round, she was quite confused – I seemed calm and in control, but the contractions were every three minutes!

We decided we should go to the hospital just to check how things were progressing. It took twenty-five minutes to get me to the car, as I kept stopping to breathe and visualise! When we got to the hospital, they told my husband not to get my bags, as it was too early, but that they'd check my progress anyway. Apparently, the midwife joked that it would be ages yet, took a look, and then said, 'Oh ... Feel free to start pushing!'

I was 10 cm dilated but so calm no-one believed it! During the pushing, mum and Paul used all the encouraging words I had written down. I especially remember them saying that the baby was safe and gliding through putty! After one-and-a-half hours of pushing, my daughter Amelie was born. Her heartbeat hadn't dipped once, and she was so chilled that she fell asleep. Within five hours, all three stages were complete, with no pain relief, no stitches, no screams and a happy baby!"

Claire Vowell, UK

*A man loves his sweetheart the most, his wife the best, but his mother the longest –
Irish proverb*

During the birth

- Sitting on the ball encourages a natural swaying or rotating motion of the pelvis, which helps the baby to descend.

- The ball provides perineal support without a lot of pressure.

- The ball helps keep the baby aligned in the pelvis.

- The sitting position assumed on the ball, similar to a squat, opens the pelvis, which helps the birthing process.

- Allows the partner to provide massage or counter-pressure to the back.

- With the ball placed on the bed, you can stand and lean into its softness, encouraging pelvic swaying and mobility.

- With the ball on the floor or bed, you can kneel and lean over the ball, encouraging pelvic motion, which can aid a posterior baby in turning to the correct position.

- The mother's weight is supported entirely by the ball.

- Moving on the ball helps your breathing to flow more evenly. This encourages the free expression of sound, a natural way to modify pain.

After the baby is born

- The ball provides support without excessive pressure on the perineum.

- During breastfeeding, it keeps posture correct and gently exercises the mother while nursing.

- Babies like gently bouncing when the person cuddling them is sitting on a ball.

- If you need to wind your baby, you can sit with your baby on your shoulder or knee as you gently bounce up and down on the ball. This helps your baby's digestion.

And, of course, a few months after your baby has been born, you can then go on to use the ball as a way to rebuild your muscle tone.

Before you were born I carried you under my heart. From the moment you arrived in this world until the moment I leave it, I will always carry you in my heart
– Mandy Harrison

Homeopathy

Homeopathic remedies can be invaluable during labour and will support and promote the physiological process without any harmful side effects. The remedies suggested below are very general remedies for labour, which can be used by everyone.

You can also consult a homeopath if you would like to put together a homeopathic labour kit that is specifically relevant to you as an individual. Helios have birthing kits which come with a very useful guide to the different remedies and their uses before, during and after the birth.

Homeopathic remedies are delicate. Touch them as little as possible. Shake one pill into the lid of the phial and tip it directly into your mouth. Remedies should be allowed to dissolve in your mouth and should not be taken with water or food. Discard any remedies that fall out accidentally. Store your remedies in a cool, dark, dry place.

The following remedies are recommended for general use during labour. They can be used to support the natural birth process or alongside other medication or interventions. Homeopathic remedies can also speed healing and recovery after the birth. It's a good idea to label the remedies beforehand according to their use, e.g. 'ease discomfort', 'backache', 'weepy', etc.

It usually works best if your partner takes responsibility for offering you any remedies that you may need, so that you can focus on the birthing.

Partner: Taking some time to familiarise yourself with the various remedies before labour starts will be advantageous. During the birth, you will naturally be observing her physical and emotional state carefully. If you know what each remedy is used for, then you can offer her the remedy that seems most appropriate. If she does not seem interested, she does not need a remedy at that time. Avoid disturbing the rhythm of labour, and offer her the remedy between contractions when she "emerges" and makes contact with you herself.

It's best to use only one remedy at a time, and repeat only if the symptoms persist or recur. If the remedy does not seem to help, then try a different one. If she is showing more than one relevant symptom, e.g. if she is in pain (Arnica) and exhausted (Kali Phos), then allow ten minutes or so between remedies.

People become really quite remarkable when they start thinking that they can do things. When they believe in themselves they have the first secret of success
– Norman Vincent Peale

General homeopathic remedies for use during labour

Arnica 200 – This wonderful remedy is beneficial to nearly all women in labour. It can be administered regularly throughout labour to help the muscles function properly, and to reduce exhaustion and pain.

Aconite 200 – Reduces fear, anxiety and panic. It is very helpful when labour is too fast and frightens the woman, and when contractions are overwhelming. Can be taken before labour where there is fear or anxiety about the birth.

Caulophyllum 200 – Used to promote strong, productive contractions in early labour. Useful where contractions are ineffectual, sharp, painful, and short, often concentrated in the lower abdomen and groin. Also good for weak contractions due to exhaustion in a long labour. Do not use routinely throughout labour.

Gelsemium 200 – Next best choice if Caulophyllum doesn't help with weak contractions. To be used when you are experiencing physical heaviness, heavy eyes and limbs, muscular weakness leading to trembling, and/or chilliness, and in the self-doubt phase.

A mum's experience

"Along with the Natal Hypnotherapy tools, I used homeopathy and reflexology throughout my pregnancy and labour. At 1 a.m. my contractions started, but I wasn't sure if it was Braxton Hicks. At 4 a.m. I knew it was labour. I used the MP3, TENS machine and homeopathy. At 7.30 a.m. my waters broke (I was using reflexology). We rang the hospital and they said I could stay at home until I wanted to come in.

I was delighted. When I went into hospital at 10.30 a.m. I was examined and was already 6–8 cm. I was very calm, doing my breathing ... My midwife and my husband were fantastic and very supportive. At 12.51 p.m. I gave birth to baby Leah, standing up. I was overcome with gratitude for having such a fantastic birth experience. Everything was as I had wanted it to be. Thank you."

Deanne Hood, Ireland

People with goals succeed because they know where they're going
– Earl Nightingale

Kali Carb 200 – Useful for backache labours or a posterior presentation. For chilliness after a contraction.

Kali Phos 200 – For exhaustion or low energy.

Pulsatilla 200 – For weepiness, clingyness, pleading for help. Contractions short, weak or stopped entirely.

[1] Touch Research Institute, http://www6.miami.edu/touch-research/Research.html.

[2] Pert, C., *Molecules of Emotion*, Simon & Schuster, 1st edition (17 February 1999).

[3] "Waterbirths: a comparative study. A prospective study on more than 2,000 waterbirths", Geissbuhler V., Eberhard J., Clinic for Obstetrics and Gynecology, Thurgauisches Kantonsspital, Frauenfeld, Switzerland. Fetal Diagn Ther 2000 Sep–Oct;15(5):291–300.
"A retrospective comparison of water births and conventional vaginal deliveries". *Eur J Obstet Gynecol Reprod Biol* 2000 Jul;91(1):15–20, Otigbah C. M., Dhanjal M. K., Harmsworth G., Chard T.

[4] "The Effects of Whirlpool Baths in Labor: A Randomized, Controlled Trial", Janet Rush, RN, BScN, MHSc, Susan Burlock, RN, Kim Lambert, RN, Margot Loosley-Millman, BSc, MD, PhD, FRcS(C), Brian Hutchison MD, MSc, CCfc Murray Enkin MD, FRCS(C), FSOG(C), *Birth*, Volume 23 Issue 3, Pages 136–143, 2 April 2007.

[5] Odent, M, *Birth and the Family* Journal (Vol. 8).

[6] Balaskas, J., 2004, *The Water Birth Book*, Thorsons.

[7] Münstedt K., Schroter C., Brüggmann D., Tinneberg H. R., von Georgi R. "Use of complementary and alternative medicine in departments of obstetrics in Germany". *Forsch Komplementmed*. 2009 Apr;16(2):111–6. Epub 3 April 2009.
Smith C. A., Collins C. T., Cyna A. M., Crowther C. A. "Complementary and alternative therapies for pain management in labour". Cochrane Database Syst Rev. 2003;(2):CD003521. Review.
Burns E., Blamey C., Ersser S. J., Lloyd A. J., Barnetson L. "The use of aromatherapy in intrapartum midwifery practice: an observational study". *Complement Ther Nurs Midwifery*. 2000 Feb;6(1):33–4.
Burns E. E., Blamey C., Ersser S. J., Barnetson L., Lloyd A. J., "An investigation into the use of aromatherapy in intrapartum midwifery practise". *J Altern Complement Med*. 2000 Apr;6(2):141–7.
Burns E., Blamey C. "Complementary medicine. Using aromatherapy in childbirth". *Nurs Times*. 1994 Mar 2–8;90(9):54–60. No abstract available.

[8] Hibbitts M., Beckley M., 2008, *The Essential Exercise and Birth Ball Handbook*, Miracle Products ltd.

Don't be discouraged if your children reject your advice. Years later they will offer it to their own offspring – Oscar Wilde

A mum's experience

"At last I have five minutes to indulge myself by telling you the story of Henry's birth. At about 5 p.m. on Sunday evening, I was having a long and lazy siesta, listening to my track. I felt a mild contraction, but knew straight away that the labour was starting.

I had the most amazing feeling of strength and power as I lay there, knowing what was going to happen — I felt so ready and so happy that I smiled to myself.

Ollie came home a little later and I told him that the baby was coming. We went for a walk to a friend's house, had a glass of wine and two paracetamol(!), and arranged childcare for the night. The lovely midwife that I had arranged to have was free and so phoned the unit on my behalf. She managed to get the overstretched coordinator to agree to let me have a home birth, even though it was officially 'too early'.

The midwife was sent to check up on where we lived and meet us. We had not met her before, but she seemed really lovely and was thrilled to hear I was using natal Hypnotherapy as she knew Maggie and had attended Maggie's second and third births as a student. We couldn't believe it — how fab!

Jen went away again as I decided it was time to take myself off to bed. I spent time listening to the birth preparation track in the dark, under my duvet, where I had done
all the practising. It felt so amazing. I was so happy — with every contraction I was allowing my body to do its thing, and it was working! It felt like the most natural thing in the world, and I was enjoying it.

Ollie came to join me after a while and was able to support me in different positions, occasionally prompting me to relax my jaw, or shaking my apples! He felt so relaxed and confident — he did not worry for a single minute, and he felt that he knew what his role was. Things just came naturally to him, too.

Anna, my wonderful mother-in-law, was also prompting me. She reminded me to turn down the comfort dial. I didn't think that I had given the comfort dial much practice, but it was something that really helped me. I used it to get me to the end of really intense contractions.

During the early stages with each contraction I had the words 'pressure, warmth and power' just arrive in my head when I needed it - incredible stuff.

Later on I focused heavily on my body and what was happening but I didn't try to focus, it just happened. It was after he was born that I looked back and realized that it just happened like that. Ollie said that I 'just got on with it'. That is how it felt, it felt like I was able to accept what was happening to my body and go with it.

The midwife came back at about 2. 30 and at this point I decided that I needed some gas and air. I had used gas and air in my previous birth, but really didn't like the feeling it gave me, but this time felt very different as was able to be in control of it (rather than the other way round as it had felt before). My midwife arrived at about 3 am and it was about then that I had a bit of 'self doubt' and asked for pethidine. I was basically told 'nope' and asked once more (just to be sure), after which I managed to get through it with Anna and Ollie's help.

I felt my breath change and knew that the baby was making his way down and this felt really incredible. I was so happy and I knew he would be here soon. I heard the music change to the bit where the baby comes and told Ollie and Anna (up until now I hadn't really done much talking). My waters broke at the last minute and little Henry was born very easily and quickly at 4 20 am. I didn't feel any pain at all pushing him out, all I felt was pure joy!

I then had a natural third stage where the placenta came away in 6 minutes, apparently that is quick?

It couldn't have been a more perfect experience. I'm over the moon.

9 days later and I have a very happy baby, very chilled, is great at feeding, really happy to receive big sloppy snotty kisses from his big brothers and who entertains us all. I am managing the sleep thing so far and am about to get started on the post-natal CD to get some super sleep!

There is no doubt in my mind that this fabulous pregnancy and birth experience I had was because of the Natal Hypnotherapy. So thank you."

Kate Room, UK

Step 5 – Prepare your birth partner

Choosing your birth partner

For thousands of years, women gave birth in their own surroundings, with one-to-one care from loving, experienced women. Traditional midwives were simply women in the community who knew and understood birth and who provided women with love, care, support and advice during their pregnancy.

As you know, in the last 100 years, the culture of giving birth has changed dramatically, moving from home to hospitals, where in many circumstances women are no longer given one-to-one support. Instead they are cared for by midwives with whom they often have no previous relationship. Without doubt, this has had a profound impact on the level of confidence, and often on the birth outcome, that women experience.

Since the 1970s, there has been a shift towards fathers being at the birth, so that nowadays it is expected that they are present, regardless of whether they really want to, or in some cases whether they should, be there. For many, being present at the birth is a treasured and awe-inspiring event. However, for some, birth can be perceived as an ordeal which they feel obliged to attend, despite the fact that they are unsure of how they can help their partner, or of how they will cope.

Sadly, preparing fathers for birth is fairly uncommon, even today, so many go into the birthing room with no knowledge or tools to use and are just expected to know what to do. They are often scared, embarrassed and feel out of their depth. As a result, they are pumping out adrenalin (which the mother will absorb as well) and heavily rely on the medical team to "do something", often seeking additional medical intervention during labour, before the mother needs it or when it may not actually be necessary.

In light of these two factors, more and more women are seeking to reclaim their birth experience and are once again seeking support from other women, including

Did you know?

In the Sherpa community of the Himalayas, fathers attend their wives through-out labour. Mother and father are united in a joint effort.

The best portion of a good man's life is the little, nameless, unremembered acts of kindness and love – William Wordsworth

relatives and birth professionals such as doulas and independent midwives. These women can offer consistent one-to-one care, which has been clinically proven to reduce the level of intervention, shorten the length of labour, and enable the woman to have a better birth experience[1].

Planning ahead

When planning who to have at the birth, it is important that you remember that it is **your** birth and that you will benefit from feeling as relaxed and confident as possible. You have a choice, and being honest now about who you want to support you will pay off many fold.

1. Think carefully about who, and what support, you may want during the labour.

2. Have an open and honest discussion with your partner about how you feel. If either of you have any concerns, then discuss alternative options, such as having a close friend, family member or doula to provide additional support.

3. Discuss the kind of things you would, and would not, like your partner to do, the kinds of intervention that you may or may not be open to, and any fears or concerns that either of you have. By talking about these now, it will help with decision-making and avoid any misunderstandings or underlying tension during the birth.

4. Spend time together preparing for the birth by going through the exercises in this book, attending a course together, and learning and practising different techniques, such as massage, visualisation, relaxation and breathing.

Other support available

Many couples who realise that it is OK for the father not to be the sole supporter, and even not to be at the birth at all, are turning to professional birth supporters such as doulas or independent midwives.

Did you know?

For the Dinka people of the Sudan, the midwife is known as the 'geem', receiver of God's gift of a child. She is the spiritual mother of the new-born, a relationship that the child will honour throughout her life.

If you could get up the courage to begin, you have the courage to succeed
– David Viscott

Doulas

Doulas are experienced birth companions who offer emotional and practical support before, during and after the birth. A couple will meet the doula several times before labour in order to get to know each other and to discuss their hopes and concerns.

> *Did you know?*
> Research has shown that having a doula with you can dramatically increase your chance of having a natural birth.

The doula will then be with you throughout the birth, giving you her constant and focused attention. A doula is also a great support for the father, should he choose to be present at the birth, as she can help with decision-making and help him to care for his partner in the most effective way.

A doula will charge between £300 and £1500 for her services before and during the birth (regardless of how long the labour takes), although trainee doulas will charge much less. Many doulas offer a postnatal service at an hourly rate, to help you care for your baby, provide support with breastfeeding and help keep the house in order.

Independent midwives

Women who are aware of the benefits of giving birth in the comfort of their own home, and of having the constant one-to-one support of someone they have known throughout pregnancy, may choose to hire an independent midwife.

Independent midwives are fully qualified midwives who have chosen to work outside the NHS, in order to provide continuity of care and to empower mothers to have a positive birth outcome. An independent midwife will charge approximately £3,500 for the duration of your pregnancy, which includes all antenatal and postnatal care through to 28 days after the baby is born.

> *I have reached a point in my life where I understand the pain and the challenges; and my attitude is one of standing up with open arms to meet them all*
> *– Myrlie Evers*

The role of the birth partner

No matter who you choose to have at the birth with you, they will play a vital role in helping you stay focused, calm and instinctive. It is important that you have been through the ideas in this book, or those you learn on the course, so that you are all "singing from the same hymn sheet".

You are likely to find that most midwives will fully support and encourage you in your plan to have an instinctive and positive birth. However, it may occasionally be the case that labour-ward staff are sceptical about hypnosis techniques or that they do not know how to work with a woman who appears calm, relaxed and confident. So it will be the job of your partner to keep you motivated, focused and Encouraged.

Did you know?

In colonial America it was common to have the labouring woman seated on her husband's lap, he being seated in a chair. He would hold onto the woman around the top of the abdomen or under her arms.

As a male writer commented in 1882, "This position was certainly not a bad one for all parties, with the exception of the father, who in tedious cases suffered rather badly."

A mum's experience

"The techniques that both I and my husband learnt meant that we had the birth we wanted. A few times during the labour I remember shouting that I couldn't do it (self-doubt), and needed something stronger; however, my husband was fantastic and used everything that had been taught on the course. I also had a fantastic midwife, who stood back, turned lights down, and just let us get on with it, without being asked. I would recommend Natal Hypnotherapy to anyone, and in fact I have."

Alfie George Taylor, UK

It is not flesh and blood but the heart which makes us fathers and sons
– Johann Schiller

Birth "support"

Physiologically a woman needs no "support" to give birth – her body is perfectly designed to birth her baby unassisted. However, she can greatly benefit from emotional and practical support, especially when she has chosen to give birth away from familiar surroundings. Key factors which will help her relax and let go are that she feels safe and unobserved, does not feel judged, and has focused, continuous care.

Some women benefit from physical support such as massage or being held, while others may not want to be touched at all. Some mothers gain tremendous encouragement from verbal support – such as being told how well they are doing, or focused counting through each contraction – while others will find that distracting.

A woman's needs will also vary according to the different stages of labour. Often, simply having someone present in the room is enough. However, all women benefit from not having to make decisions or respond to questions, from minimal distractions, and from being in an environment where they feel safe and at ease.

A woman in labour becomes very primal, but also very vulnerable, and so is extremely receptive to the words, feelings and emotions of those around her. She will pick up on the slightest concern, change in mood or change in body language, even down to the raising of an eyebrow when having her blood pressure taken.

A good birth partner does not seek to "coach" or tell her what to do, but quietly observes and picks up on her needs and emotions, giving her the encouragement, as well as the physical and mental support, to help her relax and allow her body to birth her baby.

Acting as a gatekeeper

As the birthing partner, you may like to view your role as that of her **gatekeeper**. As you know, a birthing woman is essentially a mammal. To have the most natural and comfortable birth, there are a few basic rules, all of which revolve around keeping the higher intellectual or thinking part of the brain, the neocortex, out of the equation. As her gatekeeper, your role is to ensure that all external stimulation is kept to an absolute minimum, and to keep adrenalin out of the birthing room during the serious part of labour.

A social unit is where the father is concerned with parking space, the children with outer space, and the mother with closet space – Evan Esar

With these things in place, the mother can completely hand over to her birthing brain and body, knowing that you will be there to meet her basic needs and to ensure that she feels safe, comfortable and relaxed.

What is required of the birth partner

Use the special pages at the end of this book to make notes of the tools and techniques that you can use during the birth.

Physically: Your presence and your attention to her and her needs and feelings are the most important aspects of your support. (See Step 4, on practical skills, for more ideas.)

- Attend to her basic needs – offer her drinks (don't ask if she wants anything – just put a drink to her lips); help her to the toilet; bring her a duvet or a blanket; put a cool flannel on her face; bring her a hot-water bottle to put on her tummy.

A dad's experience

"I attended the course, as Jane felt it would be useful. To be honest, I was very sceptical and worried that it would all be a bit earth-mothery and weird. However, it was the best thing we did. It helped me to fully understand the physical as well as the emotional aspects of birth (not something I had ever thought of before); plus, all the practical exercises made me feel like I had a real role to play.

I especially liked the '3, 2, 1, relax', as I could see that just a few words and a gentle stroke could help Jane become completely relaxed.

During the labour, I used the back pressure we were shown and the 'shaking the apples' – it may seem a bit weird, but, as a sports therapist, it made so much sense and Jane seemed to really enjoy it. She seemed to get even more relaxed after I had done it. It was long and tiring, but I actually enjoyed the experience and felt that the knowledge that I had gained helped me stay calm and able to help her."

Jake Toll, UK

Each child is an adventure into a better life, an opportunity to change the old pattern and make it new – Hubert Humphrey

- Take care of all practical things – taking the bag to the car; calling relatives; bringing enough snacks and drinks for both of you; having change for the car park; filling the pool (if at home).

- Some women love to be held or massaged, while others wish to be left alone. Where and how she wants physical support may also change at different points in the birthing.

Emotionally: love, support, encouragement.

- Let her know you believe in her strength and power to give birth.

- Remind her of other challenges she has accomplished.

- Trust her to birth in the best-possible way for her, even if it is different from what you expect.

- Stay with her, encourage her, and express positive beliefs and statements.

- Your attitude and trust in her can make all the difference, because her open and vulnerable mind can be strongly influenced.

- When speaking to her, recognise that you are communicating with her "birthing mind", which is not in the ordinary everyday consciousness.

- Remember that the key to managing each contraction is breathing and relaxation. Breathe with her and encourage her to use her relaxation trigger, such as saying, "3, 2, 1, relax".

- Use the visualisations she has included in her hypnosis script. Always gauge from her if she is enjoying them and if she is finding them useful. Every now and again, check that she is comfortable with your pace, timing, and phrasing, to ensure that you are in synchrony with her. It is so important not to feel offended or upset if she does not find your help useful at any given point.

- Speak slowly; pause for a few seconds after each phrase. In general, guide her through the imagery using a soft voice, pausing between each phrase. Give her adequate time to complete each step before going on to the next.

- At times she may prefer just relaxing and breathing rhythmically, with no speaking.

It is a wise father that knows his own child – William Shakespeare

Mentally: You are the spokesman for her once in the medical environment.

- You will be the gatekeeper, protecting her environment and keeping others at bay, ensuring she can birth in her own space with quiet and privacy – remember the Baobab tree.

- Liaise directly with the medical team (see more later).

A doula's experience

"My client had decided to give birth in her local hospital, as, even though it was only four minutes from her house, it was where she felt she would feel the safest. She was birthing really well at home, and all the signs were there that she was ready to move into hospital to give birth. We had brought her birth ball, duvet, eye mask, earplugs, etc to help her stay in her own "Baobab tree".

By the time we got to the main entrance of the hospital, she was having very strong and frequent contractions – so much so that she could not really move very far at all. With each contraction, she would flop over her ball, I would throw her duvet right over her, and she would gently and quietly breathe through the contractions, completely oblivious to what was going on around her.

I have to say, though, that it was a real sight, as we were right in the middle of the two automatic doors at the main entrance of the hospital, with all kinds of people coming and going and just gaping at the sight of a large, moving duvet!

However, for my client, she had her perfect space. This happened dozens of times until we finally reached the maternity unit, where she calmly birthed her baby."

Maggie Howell, UK

I'm moved by contraries, by opposites, the strength that was my mother's eyes, the beauty of my father's hands – Judith Jamison

How to make the most of the hospital environment

Today obstetrics still focuses on the role of the doctor and this preoccupation with how best to control and master childbirth[2] *– Pam England*

Here are a few tips if you are planning a hospital birth.

In most hospitals today, giving birth is a fairly medicalised and institutionalised event, with rules, time constraints, guidelines and procedures. These things, as well as the influence of "white coat syndrome", can often interfere with a woman's natural birthing rhythm and so cause adrenalin "blips" and an increase in fears and concerns. As we have seen, this can then interfere with the natural process of birth and can often lead to an increased need for medical intervention, which would not have been necessary had the mother been left to birth in her own space and time.

Therefore, one of the first tips is to stay at home as long as possible – more people get to hospital too soon than too late. The surest way **not** to have an instinctive birth is to be surrounded with adrenalin-inducing factors and to be frustrated by a long stay in hospital, with all its routines, guidelines and processes.

A mum's experience

"The course was an excellent way for my husband and I to prepare for our second baby. It helped me overcome some of the concerns I had in relation to the birth, and James felt he was given the techniques to take a very active role in my labour – he supported me (using the skills learnt at the course) through each contraction, which helped me manage each one calmly and minimised the pain, for example by encouraging me to relax the shoulders and the jaw. This was invaluable during my contractions.

James and I thoroughly enjoyed the course. It was a really great two days – very informative and helpful, yet objective. It was also a great way for us both to bond before the birth of Olivia."

Rosalind Vicherman, UK

I don't care how poor a man is; if he has family, he's rich
– Dan Wilcox and Thad Mumford

By choosing to give birth in a low-risk birthing unit, the midwives are more geared up to support instinctive birthing, as the environment is often calmer and more relaxed than on a hospital labour ward.

Wherever you choose to give birth, there are many things you can do to ensure that you create the right environment and space to birth instinctively.

> *Did you know?*
>
> Among the peoples of the Yucatan peninsula, the father is expected to support the birthing mother. This rule is quite stringent, and absent fathers are blamed for poor birth outcomes.

1. **Privacy**: Keep the number of people in the room to a minimum. A birthing mother should not feel observed (and this includes using cameras, videos and foetal monitors), as this increases her level of anxiety, inhibitions, and expectation to "perform".

   Think about it from another angle: how easy would it be for you to fall asleep knowing people are watching you? For this reason, many birthing women choose to spend time in the shower or the toilet, as it gives them privacy.

2. **Safety**: As far as possible, reduce all potential concerns and anxieties. Keep the adrenalin production to a minimum.

3. **Low lights**: As with all mammals, a birthing mother is more likely to feel safe and private if the lights are dimmed.

4. **Language**: In the serious phase of labour, keep speaking (especially questions) to a minimum. It is the use of language which stimulates the neocortex the most. If other people in the room want to speak, ask them to do so outside the room. It is even a good idea to ask for silence when she is having a contraction, so that she is completely undisturbed by any talking.

5. **Warmth**: The temperature is also important. Many hospitals have air conditioning in the summer, so bring your own blanket or duvet. The temperature is especially important after the baby is born – keep them both really warm.

> *Your children are not your children. They are the sons and daughters of Life's longing for itself – Kahlil Gibran*

Many women who use Natal Hypnotherapy are almost unaware of their surroundings and, as they have given themselves suggestions on how to deal with adrenalin-inducing factors, are able to stay calm and focused no matter what is going on around them.

When you meet the midwives who will be supporting you both, it is essential that you explain that you are using Natal Hypnotherapy, that you are keen to have an instinctive birth, and that you want to work with them to make sure all your needs are met. You can explain that she would like to have the room as quiet as possible, with the lights turned off and the door closed.

All midwives have the woman's interest at heart and have positive intentions behind everything they do. However, midwives today have a tough job, and are bound by their procedures, time constraints and guidelines. On the whole, they are used to caring for mothers who are fearful, tense and looking to them to help, and so they may offer intervention and pain relief as a matter of course. However, given the choice, the majority of midwives would dearly love for all women to have the skills that you will have, as well as the right environmental conditions to birth instinctively.

It is essential that you develop a good rapport with them and that you remain calm and friendly whilst still assertive in your role of maintaining the mother's calm, quiet birthing space. Always remember that they are there to help if help is truly needed.

Countless midwives have commented on how wonderful births have been with women Using Natal Hypnotherapy and how it has reminded them of why they became a midwife. So, you may like to see part of your role as a wonderful opportunity to inspire and motivate midwives who may be stressed, tired and de motivated.

What should you do if the mother appears to be tensing up?

By the time she is in serious labour, you will be aware of her birthing patterns – the way she breathes, her coping strategies, and so on. For much of the time, your role will simply be to be with her and to step in when she needs a drink, a massage, a few words, a hug, and so on.

By being so in tune with her, you will also become aware if her manner and disposition seem to change suddenly. This is usually a sign that she is having an "adrenalin blip" or is entering the self-doubt phase. It may be that her breathing changes, or that her body becomes more tense or she becomes more vocal. This can be due to physical changes in the birthing –

One of the obvious facts about grown-ups to a child is that they have forgotten what it is to be a child – Randell Jarrell

for example, the contraction after her waters break can be significantly more intense – or it can be emotional, such as a fear or concern has appeared.

If this happens, here are a few things you can do:

- Ask her what has just gone through her mind. Quite often it is a thought which has triggered off the fear and adrenalin. Encourage her to talk about the fears between contractions. Do not expect to solve it for her – she may just want you to listen and hear her fears, rather than offer her advice or encouragement.

- Take her through a letting-go and fear-release exercise (See Step 1 – Overcoming Fear - there is also a download that will help you let go of fear)

- If you can remove the source of her fear or disturbance, then do so. She may not like the midwife, or may be disturbed by people coming in and out. You can always ask to change midwives or ask for people to knock and then wait to be invited in.

- Provide more privacy – ask people to leave the room. Think of the Baobab tree.

- Avoid unnecessary procedures, such as vaginal examinations or over-monitoring of the baby, until she has got back into her "zone".

- Change the environment – dim lights, and provide warmth and quiet.

Remember that an adrenalin blip usually lasts just a short while; her body will then get rid of the adrenalin through the urine. Therefore, it is a good idea to allow a short time for adrenalin to decrease and endorphins and oxytocin to increase, before suggesting that she go for a wee.

To help her get over her adrenalin blip, remember to:

1. Shake the apples (see Step 4).

2. Change position, go for a wee, move around a little (see Step 4).

3. Use your triggers for deep relaxation, such as '3, 2, 1, relax' (see Step 3).

What should you do if it feels like the medical team are taking over?

Once in the hospital environment, if things are taking longer than the norm, the maternity and medical teams can be very persuasive and in some cases even forceful. Remember that they are used to dealing with scared, medicated mothers, and years of conveyor-belt

Children think not of what is past, nor of what is to come, but enjoy the present time, which few of us do – Jean de la Bruyère

intervention. Nine times out of ten, proposed intervention is not a real emergency and is often more to do with processes, timing and resources than with anything else (see chapter on Maternity guidelines – it's your choice).

So, what should you do if a midwife or doctor begins putting pressure on you both to "move things along"?

Whatever happens, it is vital to stay calm and cordial and never to generate hostility, as a birthing woman simply cannot relax in a hostile environment. Always remember that many "interventions" are based on protocol or procedures and not on a precise evaluation of your individual circumstances.

Did you know?

In the nineteenth century, American women chose to have midwives, relatives or friends attend their birth – doctors were typically mistrusted and consulted only in desperate cases.

The definition of a protocol is "the accepted code of behaviour in a particular situation"[3].

It is a way of doing things in a given institution or situation. However, it is always interesting to note that many hospitals have different protocols and that these frequently change. Therefore, they are simply guidelines and are not written in stone or based on conclusive evidence.

Ask yourself this: what is more important – having the best-possible birth for you as individuals, or following hospital processes and protocols?

Imagine that a midwife has entered the room and looked at the clock (again) and is commenting on the fact that things seem to be going slowly and suggesting that you should perhaps discuss ways to speed things along.

Firstly, stay calm, and ask the following questions:

- Is she in any danger?

- Is our baby in any danger?

If the answer is no, then simply smile, nod, and say,

> *"In that case, why do we need to rush? Could you please leave us for half an hour? We have a few things we would like to do. We can talk then."*

A child should not be denied a balloon because an adult knows that sooner or later it will burst – Marcelene Cox

In the majority of cases, that will be absolutely fine. If, however, there is increased pressure, then it is OK for the birth partner to use their BRAINS by asking the following questions to help them to make a decision:

- B – What are the Benefits? How will this be helpful?
- R – What are the Risks? What are the advantages and disadvantages?
- A – What are the Alternatives? This may be routine treatment, but what other approaches are there?
- I – What does your Instinct tell you?
- N – What if we do Nothing? Why must this be done now? What might happen if we wait another half an hour or an hour?
- S - Smile

If you are still not sure, you have the right to ask for a second opinion.

Tip: It is useful to write these onto a small card to take in with you, so that you have the questions as a prompt just in case.

Of course, it goes without saying that if there appears to be a strong and conclusive reason for intervention, then that is the time to say thank you to the amazing medical support that we do have. We are extremely blessed to have such wonderful medical support when it is truly necessary, and which ultimately saves lives.

---

[1] The obstetrical and postpartum benefits of continuous support during childbirth.
Scott K. D., Klaus P. H., Klaus M. H. J Women's Health Gend Based Med 1999 Dec;8(10):1257–64 Division of Public Health, County of Sonoma Department of Health Services, Santa Rosa, California 95404, USA.
Effects of psychosocial support during labour and childbirth on breastfeeding, medical interventions, and mothers' wellbeing in a Mexican public hospital: a randomised clinical trial.
Langer A., Campero L., Garcia C., Reynoso S. Br J Obstet Gynaecol 1998 Oct;105(10):1056–63. The Population Council, Regional Office for Latin America and the Caribbean, Colonia Coyoacan, Mexico DF,
Mexico.
Continuous emotional support during labor in a US hospital. A randomized controlled trial.
Kennell J., Klaus M., McGrath S., Robertson S., Hinkley C. JAMA 1991 May 1;265(17):2197–201. Department of Pediatrics, Case Western Reserve University, Cleveland, OH.
[2] Odent, M., 1984, Birth Reborn, Souvenir Press Ltd, London.

Loving a baby is a circular business, a kind of feedback loop. The more you give the more you get and the more you get the more you feel like giving – Penelope Leach

A mum's experience

"My contact with Natal Hypnotherapy started when I contacted Maggie Howell for an appointment to discuss wanting to become a mum and my anxieties that went with this: past worries and emotions, lack of self-belief and confidence. After some one-to-one sessions, apart from feeling on top of the world, we also conceived.

I then went on to look at what other ways Natal Hypnotherapy would be able to help us towards a more relaxed pregnancy and birth. I have never been known for my relaxed attitude, and really wanted to ensure that our baby had a relaxed mum to bring her into the world, and to be confident in my ability as a mum.

Maggie again gave me the confidence, now as mum-to-be, that I needed to believe in myself. I used Maggie's 'Birth Preparation' at night. Every time I listened to it, I had such a wonderful deep and relaxing sleep that I woke up the next morning feeling ready for anything! Near the end of my pregnancy, if I felt myself getting tired or anxious, I would take myself away and put the troack on and relax – it worked marvels!

Natal Hypnotherapy were running a two-day Birth Preparation course, which both myself and my husband attended. Never have two days been better spent! The weekend started by discussing the totally natural event of birthing, and how fear can play a big part in increased pain and complications. The practitioner takes you through some relaxation and visualisation methods. We also found it very helpful as a couple to join together to enjoy the experience and share one another's feelings and fears. It was particularly useful for my husband, as he was a little uneasy as to how he would be able to play a part and be of use during the birth. The course helped him realise that he could and would play a pivotal role and be able to join in the whole experience far more than he expected.

We had been attending the NHS classes, which in themselves were very helpful, but the two days we spent on the Natal Hypnotherapy course were full of helpful hints, tips and information that we were not aware of, in particular the various phases that labour and birth send you through. Being a first-time mum, you do not know what to expect; most of the time you are told of 38-hour labours, traumas, excruciating pain, etc, all of which scared me to the point that I wondered what I had done! However, learning about the phases, such as 'self-doubt', really helped us, and when it came to the labour, I knew what to expect and how to cope with it.

At the end of the course, we drafted our own birthing script: what we would do, our visualisation tactics, our special triggers, etc. We went away feeling so excited and waiting for the special day instead of dreading it! Before the course, I felt I would never survive childbirth (a common fear, I now understand), but after the two days I felt empowered and completely able.

Our due date was 22 December. All along, I had said I didn't want a 25 or 26 December birth date; however, Christmas Day morning at home I had my show. I was very relaxed and not at all panicked, which I had expected. So, we got the Christmas dinner on, determined to enjoy a good meal before going to hospital. After my show, I felt no real discomfort, just some twinges. Later on, around 8 p.m., my contractions started: slight at first, then becoming more uncomfortable. I found walking around the house very helpful, and swaying seemed to ease the pain.

We had our visualisation worked through. We were walking up a particular hill from a past holiday and coming back down the other side as the contraction subsided. The contractions were lasting ten seconds, five of which were going up the hill, the other five coming down. My husband would be behind me during this time, counting with me and talking to me.

We carried on with this for a while, managing to grab Christmas telly along the way! I wanted to stay at home for as long as we felt comfortable. However, by 2 a.m. my contractions were coming much faster (every two minutes), and so we felt it was time. The contractions were still only lasting ten seconds.* On the way to the hospital, we continued with our hill climbing!

It was a strange experience entering the hospital. Prior to the course, I couldn't wait to get to the hospital, with all the medical support, but, after, I felt confident that we could manage this ourselves, and that I did not need them in the way I had thought. However, they were very good, and once they realised that we had our own ideas of how we wanted to experience the birth, they were very understanding.

We were left to our own devices, being checked pretty much every four hours. We were very relaxed: walking around, walking the hill, chatting, and listening to our music. As the labour developed, I did find myself becoming increasingly tired, so I eventually lay on the bed, on my side, which I found very comfortable. I did use some gas and air towards the end, but felt that this didn't overly help, and merely seemed to shorten my contractions from ten to seven seconds.

In between contractions, I would calm myself and count each one as a positive step towards meeting our baby, instead of dreading the pain. I found myself falling into a deep sleep between each contraction. It felt like I was asleep for hours*, but by now it was only a couple of minutes.

When we had arrived at the hospital, I was 5 cm dilated, but after four hours I was only 6 cm. This was because our baby had moved slightly and was now at the wrong angle. There was then discussion about preparing me for a C-section, something that I really did not want. However, with the knowledge and confidence that my husband had, he became my 'gatekeeper' and asked whether 'either myself or the baby was in any immediate danger'. The answer was 'no', so he suggested that we wait fifteen minutes before making the decision … something I will not forget. In those fifteen minutes, our little angel moved to the correct position and started crowning! From crowning to birth it was thirty minutes – and what an unforgettable, totally amazing, emotional thirty minutes that was! I had been through my self-doubt phase, knew what it was and dealt with it, came out the other side, and gave birth to our beautiful daughter naturally and in a completely relaxed state!

She came out relaxed and chuckling, no crying, scoring 9 and then 10 on the APGAR scale! I had her against me immediately after my husband cut the cord: it was such a magical experience. No drug could match that feeling of high! The midwives left us for a while just to enjoy our new baby and the whole experience.

My labour was just twelve hours, relatively pain-free and so very relaxed – something I felt I could never achieve. Our midwives were great and very open to our own methods. They enjoyed the whole experience, too! They had never had such a relaxed birth and couldn't believe how relaxed baby was too. We were welcomed with a card from them when we got home, thanking us for 'an amazing birth'.

We strongly believe our completely amazing experience was thanks to what we learned from Natal Hypnotherapy, guiding us through our fears and lack of confidence, to make us know that we could do it and would be good at it! We are now enjoying our beautiful, relaxed daughter in a completely different way than we expected!"

Alison Spouncer, UK

* These are classic signs of time distortion. Her perception of time was completely distorted in her favour – contractions seemed like only ten seconds, and she had all the time she needed to rest between contractions.

Chapter 10 – Maternity guidelines – It's your choice

Birth in our modern maternity system has moved a long way from the way women instinctively gave birth. Good nutrition, better sanitation, better health and good antenatal care has meant that birth on the whole is safer for both the mother and the baby. In cases of true emergencies we have a first-class medical system in place to ensure that women and babies are given the best-possible care. For example, prior to antenatal scans, if a woman's placenta were lying across her cervix, then it would have meant almost certain death in childbirth. In the very rare circumstances that this happens today, women are given a life-saving Caesarean section.

However, as we explored at the beginning of this book, the increasing medicalisation and "industrialisation" of birth has led to many guidelines and procedures being put in place by hospitals as part of their routine care. Unfortunately, this can often lead to the individuality of each case being overlooked and a blanket approach being used regardless of a particular woman's circumstances. These procedures, or what are now more commonly referred to as guidelines, are supposed to be reviewed every five years using the latest evidence-based research; however, changes may or may not occur based on the views and practices of the leading medical practitioners. In addition, many guidelines will also differ between each hospital, area and even country.

I recently went to an international midwifery conference at which over forty countries were represented. It was astounding how guidelines and procedures differed between countries; for example, in Greenland epidurals are very unusual – around 8% – while in some hospitals in the US the rate is over 90%. In some countries, the due date is worked out based on the date of your last period, as in the UK, and you are given an actual date, whereas in other countries you are given a month in which you are due.

Not that long ago, performing an episiotomy was the norm in this country; now, they are no longer performed as routine, as policies were updated based on the latest available research. Within the UK, the timing and rate of induction varies enormously, with some hospitals routinely inducing at ten days over, some at fourteen days over, and some not having any time-related protocol. What does that tell you? This example shows that there is no hard-and-fast rule about when a woman should, or should not, be induced.

All children wear the sign "I want to be important NOW". Many of our juvenile - delinquency problems arise because nobody reads the signs – Dan Pursuit

The point behind this is that, for many women, the medical teams supporting them lead them to believe that these guidelines and procedures are based on non-questionable clinical evidence, and in some cases are even compulsory, with many women feeling like they should be followed without question. Quite often, the full pros and cons are not given, and in some cases women are not even asked for their consent, such as in the administration of syntometrine after the baby is born. This should not happen and is effectively assault.

It should be noted that there is a changing agenda in maternity services to one of fully informed choice and that the NCT is helping to change the medical-driven approach to childbirth. However, that may not yet have filtered through to the place you plan to birth your baby. If you are to allow your body to have the best-possible chance to give birth instinctively and intuitively, it is important to make decisions about any intervention based on your personal circumstances and wishes, and not just because it is your hospital's guidelines. To help you make some of the decisions you may have to face, here is the other side to a few of the most common guidelines and the other options available to you.

Induction

On average, one in five women in the UK begin their birth journey by being given synthetic hormones which are not their own. When a woman is induced, the synthetic hormones will produce the desired physical activity, i.e. stimulating contractions in which the uterine muscles flex and release, which in many cases can often be brought on very quickly and with artificially increased force. For a woman whose body is not really ready to give birth, induction can also be a long, drawn-out process which may take several days, making her labour long and tiring. As a result, the levels of discomfort are considerably higher than when the body is allowed to gradually build up the strength of contractions.

In addition, the synthetic hormones do not stimulate the body to produce the same levels of complementary hormones, such as endorphins and relaxin, and so the delicate cocktail of hormones is severely disrupted. As a result, the experience can be far more painful and more difficult for both mum and baby. In addition, a labour which is induced is more likely to need additional intervention, such as stronger pain relief[1], and subsequently instrumental delivery (although there is no evidence that it increases the risk of a Caesarean section[2]).

In spite of this, the number of women being induced has been rising steadily over the last twenty years, even though the World Health Organisation recommends that no more than 10% of women should be induced.

Children need love, especially when they do not deserve it – Harold Hulberry

Of course, in certain cases induction can be a lifesaver. However, it is estimated that only 3% of pregnancies will result in a medical reason to be induced. Therefore, the majority of women end up with routine inductions, which are carried out purely based on time factors, impatience and resourcing, as opposed to being done for a sound medical reason. In a recent audit at Aberdeen University, in more than a quarter of cases of more than 17,000 births, researchers could not find a medical or other explanation for induction.[3]

Even though the median length of pregnancies in healthy first-time mothers is 41 weeks[4], women are being offered induction at any time from 40 weeks onwards. The irony is that the due date given to women is based on the assumption that all women are the same, that they all have the same 28-day cycle and that their genetic disposition is the same. However, all women are unique and the duration of their pregnancy will be specific to them.

By assuming that all women are the same, the guideline in many hospitals is that women will be offered induction at a certain number of days past their due date. Again, it is ironic that different hospitals will have different guidelines – some will induce at term plus 7 (41 weeks), some at term plus 10, and some have no time-based guideline at all!

The hospital whose care I was under for my first baby only carried out inductions on a Thursday, which could mean term plus 5 or term plus 12. It must be pointed out that there appears to be no hard evidence to suggest that any one of these is the "correct" time to be induced. In fact, there is no sound research which supports routine induction at any point in pregnancy.

However, in spite of this, a large number of women are being offered routine induction when there is no medical reason and, therefore, their babies are being forced to be born when they are not ready to be born. This in turn can lead to a cascade of intervention[5], additional risks and foetal distress[6], as the body's natural hormones are not able to be released, resulting in the need for further "support".

Research has also shown that routine induction of labour for reasons such as a suspected "large" baby, or for women whose waters have broken but who have not gone into spontaneous labour within 48 hours, produces no benefits but increases the likelihood of Caesarean section[7].

Level with your child by being honest. Nobody spots a phony quicker than a child
– Mary MacCracken

So what can you do if you are being offered induction?

1.   Routine checks.

One of the first things to do is ask for routine checks to be made on a regular basis to ensure that you and your baby are both in a good condition.

According to the NICE guidelines on induction of labour[8], if you choose not to be induced then you should be offered:

- Twice-weekly checks of your baby's heartbeat using a piece of equipment called an electronic foetal-heart-rate monitor.

- A single ultrasound test to check the depth of amniotic fluid (or "waters") surrounding your baby.

The reason for this is that, as you reach the end of your pregnancy, your placenta will begin to slow down, and one of the first signs that it is slowing down a bit too much is that it will not produce as much amniotic fluid around the baby. This can be checked by an ultrasound scan. If those factors are all OK, then there is no reason to be induced. You can continue to be monitored in this way every few days until you go into labour naturally.

2. Patience.

From the first appointment with your midwife you will be given a "due date". This date will almost be stamped on your forehead and will be asked of you hundreds of times during your pregnancy. As a result, so much expectation is built up around this date and your mind becomes focused on the birth happening around this time. It can therefore feel like a considerable let-down when that date comes and goes. When you have set your mind and heart on the birth happening on a specific date, other emotions can come into play such as impatience, disappointment, frustration, and so on. For many women, induction can seem like an "easy" way to have their baby now!

However, the best thing you can do for you and your baby is to wait. Your baby knows when it is ready to be born and your body will respond as soon as the time is right. Just like an apple falling from a tree – it will only fall when it is truly ripe.

Never help a child with a task at which he feels he can succeed
– Maria Montessori

A mum's experience

"I am an English woman living in France, and I had a lot of concerns about giving birth in France, as childbirth tends to be highly medicalised. The vast majority of women opt for epidurals, and no other methods of pain relief were available at my hospital – not even gas and air. This was somewhat daunting for someone like me, who has what I consider a low pain threshold; however, I really wanted to avoid an epidural if possible. At my antenatal classes, the prevailing sentiment I found amongst fellow women in the classes was one of fear. Two months before the birth I felt very afraid, and I was determined to overcome this. An Internet search led me to Natal Hypnotherapy and I listened to it as often as I could. The most immediate benefit was the reduction of fear I felt in the last weeks of pregnancy. I learned to trust my body and enjoy those last precious weeks. That cannot be understated.

Unfortunately, I had to be induced and was started on an oxytocin drip, but this did not stimulate strong contractions, so the midwife broke my waters, which started full contractions. I used the techniques I had learnt throughout labour and found that I could manage quite well. I also used homeopathy, and had a lot of support from my husband. I was thrilled that I progressed to full dilation very quickly, just as the track said could happen. There came one point when I felt very uncomfortable and asked if the anaesthetist could come to give an epidural, but the midwife said on examination that I was fully dilated and could start pushing.

She was so encouraging and said that the most difficult part was over, and, with my husband cheering me on, the final stage passed very quickly. Our beautiful daughter Emilie was born seven hours after the onset of contractions! I was over the moon that things went so well and felt so elated after the birth. I owe all this to the Natal Hypnotherapy. I can't thank you enough for that."

Karen Dequatre Cheeseman, France

It is better to bind your children to you by a feeling of respect and by gentleness, than by fear – Terence

3. Natural methods of induction.

    If you are really keen to help your baby get ready for birth, there are some things you can do which will not harm you or your baby and may just help to trigger off the birth. However, you must remember that your baby will only be born when it is ready, and no amount of the following will bring labour on artificially.

- Walking – the more you can move around, go up and down stairs, walk up hills, etc, the more your pelvis is moving and so the more your baby's head will put pressure on the part of the cervix which can stimulate oxytocin production.

- Nipple stimulation – as we have already seen, the whole process of reproduction is closely linked. The hormones released when you are physically aroused, or during love-making, are similar to the hormones released during the birth. Therefore, nipple or clitoral stimulation will release oxytocin, which in turn can lead to the uterus beginning to contract. However, this will need to be done for some time for it to be effective!

- Making love – again, during love-making and especially during orgasm for a woman, the release of oxytocin takes place. In addition, semen contains prostaglandins, a substance which ripens, i.e. softens and stretches, the cervix.

- Sweeping the membranes – this has been a practice used by midwives for a long time. It involves inserting two fingers just inside the cervical opening, and then making a turning movement, gently separating the membranes from the cervix. This stimulation is believed to agitate or stimulate the uterus to contract and releases endogenous hormones and prostaglandins. However, little clinical evidence exists to indicate the success or otherwise of this procedure.

- Evening primrose oil – the oil contains GLA (gamma-linolenic acid), which helps the body to make prostaglandins – these soften the cervix and so help the uterus begin to contract. Take three capsules a day only once you have gone beyond your due date.

- Caulophyllum – homeopathic remedy. Only take this remedy once you are at least a week overdue, as it is believed to help stimulate contractions – it can also be taken during labour for contractions which are slow and do not appear to be very productive.

- Acupuncture – the mechanism for acupuncture induction is believed to involve stimulation of the uterus through hormonal changes or direct nerve stimulation,

The heart of a mother is a deep abyss at the bottom of which you will always find forgiveness – Honoré de Balzac

and research has shown that it can be successful in bringing about contractions[9]. The first records of acupuncture being used for induction of labour come from the Jin Dynasty (AD 265 - 420)[10].

Having said all of this, if there is a true medical reason that your baby needs to be induced, then that is the time to be thankful that we have such a wonderful medical support system which can help save lives. It is also useful to point out that many women who have been induced have gone on to have drug-free vaginal births and that all the techniques in this book can still be used with positive effect.

A mum's experience

"Having succumbed to an epidural with my first baby, I wanted to do things differently this time. I learnt about Natal Hypnotherapy on a birth professionals' study day and it seemed a natural choice to help me prepare for the birth of my second baby.

My son was born eight days after his due date. I was using the the track every day and didn't feel stressed or impatient at all when my due date came and went.

I woke up in the early hours with contractions every two minutes. I put on my TENS machine and got ready to go to the hospital. When we arrived on the labour ward the birthing pool was ready. I removed my TENS machine and got straight into the warm and relaxing water. Two-and-a-half hours later our beautiful son was born, weighing 8 lbs 11 oz.

After a lovely cuddle we got out of the water and had a physiological third stage with minimal bleeding. In total my labour lasted just under four hours from start to finish. Apart from TENS and water I used no pain relief or drugs and had no vaginal examinations. This birth was the most positive experience I have ever had and I know that that is due largely to these tools. Since having my son I find myself constantly recommending Natal Hypnotherapy to my pregnant friends. Thank you."

Lorna Davies, birth professional UK

The moment a child is born, the mother is also born. She never existed before. The woman existed, but the mother, never. A mother is something absolutely new – Rajneesh

"Managed" third stage

The birth of your baby does not end once your baby leaves your body. It only ends once the placenta has been released – also known as the third stage. It has now become commonplace, if not routine in most hospitals, to automatically provide a "managed third stage" – i.e., using drugs to speed up the release of the placenta, as opposed to a natural or physiological third stage in which you simply wait for your body to release the placenta.

This "managed third stage" is done by injecting an artificial hormone (syntometrine or syntocinon) into a woman as soon as her baby has been born (and sometimes even before the baby is born), to artificially contract the uterus and release the placenta. The cord is then clamped soon after, and gentle pulling of the cord is used to help release the placenta. The drug was first used to prevent heavy loss of blood or post-partum haemorrhaging, which can be very serious indeed. In times gone by, this was one of the main reasons women died in childbirth, so, when truly needed, it saves lives.

However, the administration of this drug has now become routine in many hospitals, even when there are no indications that there is potential heavy blood loss or any other medical reason for it.

A mum's experience

"I had listened to the Natal Hypnotherapy CD during my pregnancy and had been quite sceptical, so had planned on listening to it when labour began, to get me in the right frame of mind, help me relax, etc. In the end, there was no time – when I had my first contraction, I was examined and was already at 8 cm. The baby came two-and-a-half hours later, so no time for gas and air, let alone to put the CD on! But I do remember thinking to myself that I must 'turn the dial down' during some of the contractions.

I also remembered what the CD had said about relaxing my pelvic floor, letting it open out like a fan, and this helped. My baby was born healthy and well with no pain relief or medical intervention, not even for third-stage labour. Exactly as I had hoped it would be, but I had not really expected to manage it."

Charlotte J., UK

Mother's love grows by giving – Charles Lamb

This was brought home to me when a student midwife in her third year attended one of my births – she had never seen a "natural" or "physiological" third stage". In other words, she had never seen a woman allow her body to naturally finish the process of giving birth. She was so amazed at what she saw with my birth that she wrote about it as her dissertation.

Did you know?
The placenta is a very complex organ. Every enzyme known to exist in biology (except ACTH) has been found in the placenta.

So, why has it become routine?

Again, in certain circumstances, syntometrine (a combination of syntocinon – an artificial oxytocin – and ergometrine, which makes blood vessels contract, thereby reducing blood loss) can be a life-saving drug. However, in the majority of cases it is more about speed and resourcing. In other words, once the placenta is out, the birth is officially over and so support and attention can be moved to the next person.

You may be wondering why it is an issue, as, once the baby is out, it should not really matter. Well, there are several issues to consider.

The first is that, by speeding up the release of the placenta, you are interfering with the natural exchange of blood from you to your baby through the umbilical cord. Left to nature, the cord would continue pulsating; this ensures that all the blood in the cord is passed through to the baby, so that the baby is relying on oxygen both from the air and from the cord. It is like a reserve tank for the baby as they get used to the massive changes involved with using their lungs for the first time.

In addition, we are becoming increasingly aware of the amazing properties of stem cells in the cord blood, which are only produced at this time in a baby's life. It is vital that the baby receives its full quota of these stem cells.

With a managed third stage, the cord is often clamped within thirty seconds of the birth, thus stopping this important process. It is estimated that this approach deprives the baby of almost half the full amount of blood received when the process is unmanaged[11]. In addition, this reduces the amount of iron the baby receives, which can lead to infancy anaemia[12]. This knowledge goes back a long way, with Erasmus Darwin saying in 1801:

> Another thing very injurious to the child is the tying and cutting of the navel string too soon; which should always be left till the child has not only repeatedly breathed but till all pulsation in the cord ceases. As, otherwise, the child is much weaker than it ought to be, a part of the blood being left in the placenta which ought to have been in the child.[13]

One good mother is worth a hundred schoolmasters – George Herbert

The second reason you should make an informed choice about the use of this drug is the potential impact that it can have on your ability to bond and breastfeed.

As you read earlier, the few moments just after the birth of your baby are when your body produces its highest peak of the love hormone oxytocin and endorphins. The main reason for this is simple – it is to help you fall in love with your baby and for your body to initiate the breastfeeding process.

If you interfere with this process, i.e. by introducing a synthetic hormone, your body's own production of oxytocin will be reduced, which in turn can potentially lead to difficulties bonding and subsequently breastfeeding. Little research has been done in this area; however, there have been studies which have shown that routine use of syntometrine has led to an increase in difficulties breastfeeding[14].

As with any drug, there are known side effects for the mother, including nausea, vomiting, problems with breathing, high blood pressure, retained placenta and delayed onset of milk production. It has to be noted that the main side effects are from the ergometrine part of the drug[15,16,17]. For this point, it is now recommended practice in the NICE guidelines that only syntocinon be used and not syntometrine, which is combined with ergometrine.

It seems so sad that, even when a woman has followed all her instincts and has worked with her body to give birth intuitively and naturally, those precious few moments after the birth of her baby can be interfered with simply due to guidelines. As Sarah Buckley puts it:

At the time when Mother Nature prescribes awe and ecstasy, we have injections, examinations, and clamping and pulling on the cord. Instead of body heat and skin-to-skin contact, we have separation and wrapping. Where time should stand still for those eternal moments of first contact, as mother and baby fall deeply in love, we have haste to deliver the placenta and clean up for the next 'case'.[18]

What should you do if you want a natural third stage?

The first point is to discuss this with your midwife. Explain that you would like to plan for a natural third stage, but are open to changes if your birth is augmented during labour or if you have an epidural (as then the natural flow of hormones has already been disturbed). However, if those things do not occur, then you would like it to be a matter of being patient and waiting for your uterus to contract down and release the placenta.

The strength of motherhood is greater than natural laws – Barbara Kingsolver

This can take anything from ten minutes to a couple of hours. You can say that you are happy to adopt a wait-and-see approach, so that you allow the cord to stop pulsating and the uterus to begin to contract. However, if there are any signs of heavy blood loss, you are happy to have the syntocinon then (it only takes about two minutes to work).

Remember that your body does actually know what to do, and that given the right conditions, i.e. that you are not flat on your back, you are skin to skin with your baby, your baby begins to suckle, you are warm and feel safe and relaxed, and so on, the oxytocin will trigger off all the things necessary to release the placenta safely and bring the birth process to its natural end.

Concerns over having a "big baby"

Many women are often told, based on an ultrasound scan, that they are likely to have a "big baby". This can lead to concerns and fears over whether the birth will be more difficult or even possible at all.

The first point to remember is that big babies do not necessarily lead to harder or more difficult births. In some cases, if a baby has a higher birth weight, the birth can actually be quicker and easier, as it is the pressure and weight on the cervix that helps the cervix to open and dilate. Remember that the more gravity and weight there is on the cervix, the more stimulation of the tiny hormone receptors to produce the wonderful oxytocin which makes the contractions even more effective. I have heard so many stories of women who have actually found the births of their heavier babies easier than those of their lighter babies.

Secondly, ultrasound scans are notoriously wrong when it comes to measuring the baby's birth weight accurately, often overestimating the weight. For example, one study found that the estimated weight was heavier than the actual birth weight in 66 out of 86 women studied (77%).[19]

In diabetic pregnancies, it has been demonstrated that ultrasound measurements are not more accurate than clinical examination to identify high-birth-weight babies[20]. This led to the memorable title of an editorial of the *British Journal of Obstetrics and Gynaecology*: 'Guess the weight of the baby'[21].

A special UK government report[22] concluded that ultrasound estimation of foetal weight was **NOT** recommended where a large baby was suspected, because

When you are a mother, you are never really alone in your thoughts. A mother always has to think twice, once for herself and once for her child – Sophia Loren

The inaccuracy of ultrasound estimates has been well documented. Indeed, it is possible that estimating foetal weight by late ultrasound may do more harm than good by increasing intervention rates (p. 47).

The best advice is that, if you are told you may have a "big baby", you should ask for a couple of opinions from experienced midwives; if they all agree that the baby will be large, then discuss the steps you can take to help yourself during the birth. Obviously, you need to assess your own situation, i.e. your size and the size of your baby's father; however, by nature, your body would not grow a baby that it was not capable of giving birth to.

You may be urged to have an early induction (see previous section) or a Caesarean section. However, both of these bring additional risks, and the evidence does not suggest that they improve the outcome.

If you are concerned that you are going to have a big baby, then there are plenty of things that you can do to help yourself during the labour, such as keeping active during the labour, avoiding lying on your back, avoiding synthetic hormones or drugs which interfere with your body's natural flow of labour and are more likely to lead to problems[23], and of course staying as relaxed and calm as possible.

As one of the main concerns for women having "big babies" is that the head and shoulders may need a little help passing through the pelvis, discuss with your midwives the techniques they use if the baby needs a little help. These may include the McRoberts manoeuvre (lying on your back with your knees up by your ears to open the pelvis) and the Gaskin manoeuvre (where you turn over from the lying-down position to get onto all fours and then turn over again). It is even helpful to practise them in advance so that you know what to expect.

If people comment on the size of your bump or think you are going to have a big baby, you can simply say, "Yeah, it is great, isn't it – it shows how brilliant my body has been so far in producing such a strong and healthy baby!"

---

[1] Vernon, David, 2005, *Having a Great Birth in Australia,* Australian College of Midwives, ISBN 0-9751674-3-X.

[2] Yeast, John D., "Induction of labor and the relationship to Caesarean delivery: A review of 7001 consecutive inductions", March 1999, *American Journal of Obstetrics and Gynecology.*

[3] World Health Organisation. "Appropriate technology for birth". *Lancet* 1985;2(8453)436–437.

[4] Mittendorf, R. et al., "The length of uncomplicated human gestation". Obstet Gynecol 1990:75(6):929–32.

[5] NICE guidelines – Induction of labour, July 2008, page 3. Cammu, H. et al. "Outcome after elective labour induction in nulliparous women. A matched cohort study". *Am J Obstet gynecol* 2002:186 92:240–4. Alexander J. M., McIntire D. D. and Leveno K. J. "Forty weeks and beyond: pregnancy outcomes of

Feeling fat lasts nine months, but the joy of becoming a mom lasts forever
– Nikki Dalton

[6] Goer, H., 1999, *The Thinking Woman's Guide to a Better Birth*. New York; Pedigree books, p. 228–9.

[7] Gonen, O. et al., "Induction of labour versus expectant management in macrosmoia. A randomized study", *Obstet Gynecol* 1997;89(6):913–7.

[8] http://www.nice.org.uk/guidance/CG70.

[9] Smith, C. A., 2004, "Acupuncture for induction of labour". The Cochrane Database of Systematic Reviews (1).

[10] http://www.newhm.com.au/acu_induction_2.pdf.

[11] Usher, R. et al. "The Blood Volume of the Newborn Infant and Placental Transfusion". *Acta Paediatr* 1963;52:497–512.

[12] Landau, D. B., "Hyaline membrane formation in the newborn; hematogenic shock as a possible etiologic factor". *Mo Med* 1953;50(3):183–5. Peltonen, T., "Placental transfusion--advantage and disadvantage". *Eur J Pediatr* 1981;137(2):141–6.

[13] Darwin, E. *Zoonomia or The Laws of Organic Life*. Second ed. London: J Johnson, 1796.

[14] Murphy, M, ozmidwifery RE:PS. Oxytocinon, Tue, 7 June 2005 16:16:53-0700.

[15] Prendiville W. J. P., Elbourne D., McDonald S. J. "Active versus expectant management in the third stage of labour". Cochrane Database of Systematic Reviews 2000; Issue 3. Art. No.: CD000007; DOI: 10.1002/14651858.CD000007.

[16] M. Khooshideh (M.D.), A. Shahriari (M.D.), "A comparison between oxytocin and syntometrine for preventing postpartum haemorrhage". *Journal of Reproduction and Infertility*, Volume 5, Issue 1, Year 2003, Number 17.
W. O. Chukudebelu, A. T. Marshall and J. A. Chalmers Br Med, "Use of 'Syntometrine' in the Third Stage of Labour", J. 1963 May 25; 1(5342): 1390–1391. PMCID: PMC2124037 .

[17] Sorbe, B., "Active pharmacologic management of the third stage of labor. A comparison of oxytocin and ergometrine". *Obstet Gynecol* 1978;52(6):694–7.

[18] Buckley, S. J., http://www.sarahjbuckley.com/articles/leaving-well-alone.htm.

[19] Delpapa E. H. and Mueller-Heubach E., "Pregnancy outcome following ultrasound diagnosis of macrosomia". Department of Obstetrics and Gynaecology, University of Pittsburgh, Magee-Women's Hospital, Pennsylvania.
Obstet Gynecol 1991 Sep;78(3 Pt 1):340–3.

[20] Johnstone F. D., Prescott R. J. et al., "Clinical and ultrasound prediction of macrosomia in diabetic pregnancy". *Br J Obstet Gynaecol* 1996; 103: 747–54.

[21] http://www.birthpsychology.com/primalhealth/primal10.html.

[22] *The 6th Annual CESDI report* (Confidential Enquiry into Stillbirths and Deaths in Infancy, published by UK government)
Available free online at the Confidential Enquiry into Maternal and Child Health website *(www.cemach.org.uk)*.

[23] Benedetti T. J. and Gabbe S. G., "Shoulder dystocia. A complication of fetal macrosomia and prolonged second stage of labor with midpelvic delivery", *Obstet Gynecol* 1978 Nov;52(5):526–9; Modanlou H. D., Dorchester W. L., Thorosian A. and Freeman R. K., "Macrosomia--maternal, fetal, and neonatal implications". *Obstet Gynecol* 1980 Apr;55(4):420–4.

Success is not final, failure is not fatal: it is the courage to continue that counts
– Winston Churchill

A mum's experience

"Throughout my second pregnancy I was told I had a 'big baby'. Having been through birth before, I was a bit worried about this! I kept on telling myself though that my body had made this baby and so my body could get it out! I was ten days overdue and so had to be induced. I didn't want to be, but with a toddler to think about at home and the care arrangements for her I decided it was best to get this baby out. After an overnight stay in hospital, my waters were broken and my baby arrived four hours later. She was 2 lbs heavier than my first – so a much bigger baby.

Amazingly, though, I needed no pain relief, intervention or stitches! I just went into automatic mode. I had been through it so many times with the track, I just relaxed and let my body get on with it. I am so pleased that I have had a positive birth experience after the nightmare birth of my first child. I put it solely down to the tools Id learnt and thoroughly recommend them to anyone. I wish I had listened to them before the birth of my first child."

Charlotte Belshaw, UK

A mum's experience

"I had a difficult delivery last time, as I had an allergic reaction to a drug and was not really aware of the birth experience, so I really wanted a natural birth this time. I ended up giving birth to an extremely large baby with very little difficulty and no real feeling of pain.

Throughout the labour I experienced contractions simply as tightenings or strong Braxton Hicks as long as I remained in bed and concentrated on the techniques I had leart Everyone described me as calm, happy and in control.

We decided to get ready to go to hospital once they were more frequent and stronger. There was a carnival en route and a ten-minute drive took thirty minutes, with contractions now every three minutes! But the techniques I had learnt carried me through and I was oblivious. When I was examined at 2 p.m., I was 8 cm dilated but still only felt pain when walking around.

At 3 p.m., my 10 lb 10 oz baby was born with gas and air as the only pain relief. I have no doubt I would not have managed without Natal Hypnotherapy! The staff all said I was serene and calm and at first wouldn't believe me when I told them about the length and nature of contractions. Because I was so self-contained, they even doubted their own examination.

The breathing and relaxation techniques also helped during stitching for episiotomy and this was the only time I felt real pain.

A total contrast to my first birth – thank you, thank you, thank you!"

Kate Nicholls, UK

Chapter 11 – Calmer mum, calmer baby

For many women who have used the techniques described in this book, their experience has been that the relaxation and self-hypnosis techniques have resulted not only in themselves staying calm, but also in their baby being calm, alert and relaxed.

Of course, it cannot be guaranteed that hypnosis and relaxation during pregnancy will definitely lead to your baby being calmer and more at ease; however, there is enough anecdotal evidence to suggest that it can make a big difference.

Many leading researchers and birth professionals agree that the environment *in utero* is more important to the health and well-being of a child than the environment at any other time in their life. According to Michel Odent, who has developed an amazing database of research (www.primalhealthresearch.com) on the correlation between the perinatal period and health and personality traits in later life:

> In terms of public health, it appears that nothing today is more important than the health and well-being of pregnant women. In terms of research, nothing is more important than the study of factors influencing foetal growth and foetal development.[1]

We know from many research studies that a mother's emotional state during her pregnancy can have a considerable impact on her baby – this was noted as early as 1934[2], when it was observed that there is a significant correlation between maternal stress and the baby's well-being.

However, this knowledge goes way back before the time of medicine and research:

> In many traditional societies they had an intuitive knowledge of the effects of maternal emotional states on foetal development. It was well understood that the duty of the community was to protect the emotional state of pregnant women.

Did you know?
Tsinghai women in China carry their babies with them for five years, nursing them on demand.

The greatest thing she'd learned over the years is that there's no way to be a perfect mother, but a million ways to be a good one – Author unknown

For example, I heard that in an ethnic group of Western Amazonia, they transmit the belief that people should avoid arguing with a pregnant woman, and, if by chance they start arguing, they should always make sure that the mother-to-be would have the last word.[3] (Michel Odent)

Another leading figure in research into the emotional state of pregnant women is Professor Vivette Glover, who has studied the long-term effect on children whose mothers experienced considerable stress during pregnancy. Several large-scale studies have shown that if the mother is significantly stressed or anxious while she is pregnant, the child is more likely to be anxious, have symptoms of attention deficit/hyperactivity, and have lower scores on the Bayley Mental Development index[4,5]. Much of this has been shown to be due to the reduction of blood flow to the baby in a mother who is anxious, which in turn will increase the cortisol levels in the baby[6].

BUT it is important to stress that, in much of the research, the levels of stress experienced by the women have been extremely high – it is not the "normal" kind of stress that everyone faces on a daily basis. So, if it is the case that high levels of stress are detrimental to the well-being of the baby, it must be the case that a relaxed, calm mother can only have a positive influence on the baby's well-being.

There is more and more evidence-based research being done in this area; for example, Moya and James demonstrated that babies born to mothers using hypnosis were more alert, and had better APGAR scores and more-effective respiration, than those whose mothers received anaesthesia[7]. In another study, research showed a significant positive impact on women – and their babies – who experienced relaxation using guided visualisation during week 32 of their pregnancy[8].

One of the most significant studies was carried out by Professor Glover. Women underwent short periods of relaxation each day and the findings showed that this decreased maternal anxiety, decreased their heart rate and decreased the levels of cortisol in their blood – all of which are great for the woman's baby[9]!

In another study of first-time, anxious women, the teaching of relaxation techniques again had a positive effect on the birth outcomes and the well-being of mum and baby[10]. This has also been backed up by research on the positive impact of yoga[11], relaxation

Did you know?

The Wayapo tribe of Brazil observe a "moon-long" seclusion for a mother and her new-born child, during which time they bond with each other and learn each other's shapes and smells.

The best motivation is self-motivation – Jim Rohn

therapy[12] and massage[13] on the outcomes for both mum and baby.

So, in essence, the more you can take time out during your pregnancy to relax, and of course the calmer and more instinctive your birth experience, the more likely it is that your baby will reap the rewards.

Did you know?

Mayan women who have given birth go to sleep with their babies in their arms and will not be separated until they resume normal activities after 20 days.

And so we come to the end ... Well, not really – it is just the beginning

From this point on, it is up to you – much of the research I have discussed above was based on women who experience relaxation for short periods of time only. Just imagine how much more beneficial it would be for both you and your baby to practise the techniques regularly from now on!

To bring this book to a close, I have finished off with a few heartwarming stories, showing the profound impact that relaxation, self-hypnosis and belief can have on your birth experience and on the emotional well-being of your baby.

All the reading in the world will not make it happen, so learn all you can from this book and then go and put it into practice. Only you can turn the knowledge you have gained into reality and practice. You are in control of what happens from now on – grab it with both hands and make this birth experience the best it can possibly be.

Wishing you all the very best and please let me know how you got on

Maggie Howell

maggie@natalhypnotherapy.co.uk

The greater the difficulty, the more glory in surmounting it. Skilful pilots gain their reputation from storms and tempests – Epictetus

[1] Mulder E. J., Robles de Medina P. G., Huizink A. C., Van Den Bergh B. R., Buitelaar J. K., Visser G. H., "Prenatal maternal stress: effects on pregnancy and the (unborn) child", *Early Hum Dev* 2002 Dec;70(1–2):3–14.

[2] Sontag L. W., Wallace R. F., "Preliminary report of the Fels fund". *American Journal of Diseases of Children*. 1934;48:1050–1057.

[3] http://www.wombecology.com/maternalemotional.html.

[4] O'Connor T. G., Heron J., Golding J., Beveridge M., Glover V. (2002), Maternal Antenatal Anxiety and Behavioural Problems in Early Childhood. *Brit J Psychiat* 180, 502–508.

[5] Sarker P., Bergman K., Fisk N. M., Glover V. (2006) Maternal anxiety at amniocentesis and plasma cortisol. *Prenat Diagn*. 26(6):505–9.

[6] Sarker P., Bergman K., O'Connor T. G., Glover V. (2008) Maternal antenatal anxiety and amniotic fluid cortisol and testosterone: possible implications for foetal programming. *J Neuroendocrinol*. 20;489–96.

[7] Moya F., James L. S., "Medical hypnosis for obstetrics", *JAMA* 1960; 174:2026–32a.

[8] Janet A. DiPietro, Kathleen A. Costigan, Priscilla Nelson, Edith D. Gurewitsch, and Mark L. Laudenslager, "Fetal responses to induced maternal relaxation during pregnancy", *Biol Psychol*. 2008 January; 77(1): 11–19.

[9] Teixeira J., Martin D., Prendiville O., Glover V. "The effects of acute relaxation on indices of anxiety during pregnancy". *Journal of Psychosomatic Obstetrics and Gynaecology*. 2005;26:271–276.

[10] Bastani F., Hidarnia A., Montgomery K. S., Aquilar-Vafaei M. E., Kazemnejad A. "Does relaxation education in anxious primigravid Iranian women influence adverse pregnancy outcomes? A randomized controlled trial". *Journal of Perinatal and Neonatal Nursing*. 2006;20:138–146.

[11] Narendran S., Nagarathna R., Narendran C., Gunasheela S., Nagendra H. R. R., "Efficacy of yoga on pregnancy outcome". *Journal of Alternative and Complementary Medicine*. 2005;11:237–244.

The tears of faithfulness to your beliefs cleanse your spirit to envision the road ahead. Everything is possible for the person who believes – Adlin Sinclair

A mum's experience

"When I was seven months' pregnant, my mum passed away. She had been ill for four years with terminal cancer and we knew we were living on borrowed time, but she had fought for long enough and sadly became too ill to keep battling. Two days after she died, my dad had some routine blood-test results and was soon diagnosed with leukaemia – we couldn't believe it, as he didn't even feel unwell. Five weeks later, he died. Baby Dylan was born just a week later.

It was a very emotional time – I was so sad, and trying to stay focused on the birth was impossible during the day. Each evening I would put on the relaxing birth music and was able somehow to escape and go into deep relaxation, focusing on me and the impending birth despite all the trauma around me. I had been listening to the relaxation CD for several weeks already and I believe I had trained my brain to go into relaxation mode pretty well by then.

The birth itself was strange – things were so raw, and all my held-in emotion and pain from my bereavements came out (in a roar!). During the first few hours of latent labour (which actually hurt as much as the 'real thing' by the way ...) I was great at breathing and relaxing through the contractions, keeping positive, but once I found out I was still only 3 cm dilated after 12 hours, I'm afraid I wasn't able to hold it together emotionally and ended up using primal-scream therapy instead – not quite in the birth plan! Fortunately for all concerned, the birth was 'easy' – I didn't even tear; I only had gas and air and the TENS machine, and had a beautiful baby boy four hours later. Born in his waters, he was very relaxed all the way through.

One thing I really do feel is that throughout the pregnancy, even though I used the CD with headphones, each time I played it I relaxed so much that he must have sensed this too."

Anne Mari Barker-Davies, UK

A mum's experience

"I went 12 days overdue with Group B Strep and my induction date had been booked. However, my waters broke and contractions started immediately. My midwife arrived 35 minutes later. She gave me my antibiotics for GBS and then unloaded the car, by which time she decided she needed to stay. No examination during labour, which was bliss – the midwife let me do my own thing and follow my body. She commented several times on how well I was coping with the contractions and pain. I told her about the Natal Hypnotherapy and she was very impressed.

She said she couldn't believe how calm I was! I quickly got to full dilation and then transition followed. I was coping with just TENS and breathing pretty well just before pushing, which happened completely naturally – no one told me to start pushing; my body started doing it all by itself. The midwife offered me gas and air, which I started using, although I am not sure how well it worked.

Just before pushing I remember saying to the midwife mid-contraction that I was quite enjoying this, as once the contraction started I knew it would soon be over again, if that made sense! I was only pushing for around 20 minutes, and delivered my gorgeous boy kneeling over the sofa – I pulled him through my legs to look at him and we waited for the cord to stop pulsing. His APGAR scores at birth were 10 and 10 again. He was in perfect shape and a wonderful colour.

Throughout the labour and birth his heart rate had been so stable – he was and still is a very chilled-out baby. My labour was three hours from waters breaking to delivery – not long enough for my antibiotics to be effective, so there was a bit of a wobble when we thought they may ask me and baby to transfer to hospital for 48 hours of monitoring for GBS. Aaargh – it would defeat the whole point of the home birth. Thankfully, we spoke to the paediatrician in the NICU and he was happy for us to stay at home and be visited by a midwife later in the day and for us to monitor baby at home for any signs of infection – yay! The best experience, and so, so different to my first labour and birth: 11 hours, epidural, forceps, episiotomy in theatre and threatened CS, followed by 48 hours of horrendous postnatal care.

Thanks for a wonderful experience."

Ellen Mulholland, UK

A mum's experience

"I gave birth three-and-a-half weeks early, on 3 October, with no pain relief and in only nine-and-a-half hours! I had started learning Natal Hypnotherapy from week 24 and kept insisting I would have a natural, chilled-out labour experience. Most people were sceptical, but I believed I could do it, and the support of the tracks reinforced this.

My waters broke at 9.15 p.m. on the Sunday night and I spent a calm hour getting sorted out and ready to go to hospital. I honestly thought they would check me over and send me home, as I was in no pain, but when I was examined at 10.30 p.m. I was 2–3 cm dilated, which quickly became 5 cm. The midwives and doctors found it hard to believe how calm and focused I was, even though I had to be strapped to a monitor, as baby's heart rate was rather fast. I was also put on a drip, as a Caesarean was threatened, but I knew I would have my baby naturally, so ignored their threats and focused instead on the hypnotherapy techniques (aided by the relaxation track, massage and support from birth partners, and a fabulous team of midwives and doctors.)

Baby Elise Kay was born at 8.15 a.m., assisted by ventouse, as I had been pushing for two hours and she wasn't coming out. However, I still felt totally in control and was never scared that anything would go wrong or that I couldn't cope.

I am overwhelmed by the success of this technique, and though I was fully aware of the pain, I dealt with it – in fact, my husband said I was calm the whole time and that he honestly didn't know I was in pain (apart from the time I swore loudly because I had such bad cramp!).

Anyone considering having a baby, please consider using hypnosis. I wouldn't change a thing about my experience (except maybe use the birth preparation more often).

Sadly, my baby had to go into hospital a few days later, as she was very ill – however, she was very calm, brave and focused, and amazed doctors with her progress. I can't help but think that the hypnosis techniques rubbed off on her, too – after all, a calm mum = a calm baby."

Tania Richardson, UK

A mum's experience

"My previous pregnancy ended in my daughter being stillborn at 16 weeks, so I was pretty stressed during this pregnancy and the tools really helped me to feel positive and confident and ready for anything. My husband found it useful, too, since he was a bit apprehensive and it made him much more relaxed about the labour and how he could help.

My labour really wasn't painful, although it was a very intense and powerful Experience. I didn't need any drugs and just took some gas and air at the very last stage, since I had become very anaemic and the midwives wanted to give me a Boost. In the end, the gas and air made me a bit reckless and I ended up with stitches – in many ways, I wish I hadn't taken it, but I was really very faint and it did seem to give me a second wind. I used the '3, 2, 1, relax' a lot during the labour (and I still use it now from time to time when I'm a bit tense!). I photocopied your Diagram about a peaceful birthplace and pinned it up in my bedroom so that the midwives would get the message. In the event, they were very supportive, and gave me just the right environment and encouragement I needed.

I had the music CD playing all the way through the labour and I still use it every night to put Craig to sleep. I find it helps me relax when I'm breastfeeding at night, and Craig really seems to be calm when he hears the music.

Thanks ever so much for your tools – I have already recommended them to my friends who are pregnant. My birth preparation involved a lot of reading (like Ina May Gaskin, etc) and a lot of yoga, a birth preparation class at the Birth Resource Centre in Edinburgh, and of course the Natal Hypnotherapy tracks. It was a mixture that worked well for me, and I could not have been happier with my birthing experience (except the stitches and the anaemia!).

Craig is a happy, content wee soul, and I put that all down to the relaxation during pregnancy, labour and post-birth. A calm mum and a calm baby!"

Fiona Matthews, Scotland

Appendix

Some frequently asked questions about hypnosis

Am I under someone else's control in hypnosis?

No. This idea comes from comic books, cartoons, and movies. People who believe that this happens in stage hypnosis are misinterpreting the experience. In hypnosis you are aware, and ultimately in control of everything that happens. Fundamentally, you choose to be in hypnosis and you choose whether to allow yourself to respond or not. You cannot be forced into hypnosis against your will nor can you be compelled to do anything embarrassing or objectionable. Many eminent psychological researchers have proved this fact. For instance, in the book *Modern Hypnosis*, Milton Erickson, a famous authority on hypnosis, summarises his research in precisely this area as follows:

> *The findings disclosed consistently the failure of all experimental measures to induce hypnotic subjects, in response to hypnotic suggestion, to perform acts of an objectionable character [...]. Instead of a blind, submissive, automatic, unthinking obedience and acquiescence to the hypnotist and the acceptance of carefully given suggestions and commands, the subjects demonstrated a full capacity and ability for self-protection [...].*[1]

In other words, even in the deepest levels of hypnosis, you remain in control of your responses and will not accept suggestions which are in any way objectionable to you.

Can anyone be hypnotised/practise self-hypnosis?

Yes, absolutely anyone. Entering into hypnosis is as easy as daydreaming: if you can daydream or relax your mind or fall asleep, then you can enter into hypnosis. Being able to enter into a hypnotic trance has nothing to do with your level of intelligence, strength of mind, gullibility or need to control. What can be different is the "depth" to which someone will go – some people only achieve a light trance where they are very aware of their surroundings, the voice of the therapist, etc, while others can feel as if they have slept all the way through and did not consciously hear a word that was said.

A person's ability to go into a trance can be hindered or helped by:

1. Their surroundings.
2. Feelings of trust in the therapist.
3. Ability to suspend judgment.
4. Willingness to "let go" and go with the flow.

Can I get stuck in hypnosis?

No – just as you cannot get stuck in a daydream, in meditation, or in sleep. Given time, you will either rouse yourself naturally or drift off to natural sleep; hypnosis is a temporary state of mind.

Does it mean I am weak-willed or gullible?

Definitely not – indeed, good hypnotic subjects tend to be *more* intelligent and *less* gullible than average. 'Gullibility' is a weakness of the *conscious* intellect, a form of stupidity. Hypnotic 'suggestibility' is your ability to respond to positive ideas at an experiential, emotional or unconscious level. Good suggestibility (or 'hypnotic responsiveness') is a valuable asset; indeed, real 'self-control' actually *requires* good suggestibility.

What about stage hypnosis?

Stage hypnosis is predominantly about entertainment. It has a few methods and principles in common with hypnotherapy; however, in terms of style and approach, it is obviously very different. People are chosen very carefully for their susceptibility to suggestions and their "willingness" to perform. Yes, most of the people on stage are in a hypnotic state, but they are compliant and willing participants who are "performing" the actions with awareness. In addition, they are following suggestions, as it is providing them with the opportunity to be in the spotlight and give them their few minutes of fame. There is also the strong 'belief' that they will be under someone else's control, that they will not be able to 'fight it' and that they will not remember anything afterwards – belief is a very powerful thing!

However, hypnotherapy or self-hypnosis is not about making fun of people. You will not be asked to bark like a dog, cluck like a chicken, or dance like Elvis Presley!

Is hypnotherapy a recognised form of therapy?

Yes. The British Medical Association (BMA) first recognised the genuineness of hypnosis and its therapeutic benefits back in 1892, then again following a more thorough report in 1955. The BMA recently suggested in a statement to the House of Lords that they consider hypnotherapy to be an orthodox physical and psychological treatment.

Hypnotherapy (or rather 'hypno-psychotherapy') is also officially recognised as a technique of psychotherapy by the UK Council for Psychotherapy, the principal psychotherapy organisation in the UK.

The draft NICE guidelines (National Institute of Clinical Excellence) on maternity services, published in February 2007, state that women should not be discouraged from using hypnosis as a form of pain relief during labour.

Many doctors and dentists around the world use hypnosis in their practice as well as on themselves. A dental surgeon, Dr. Victor Rausch, used hypnosis extensively in his practice; and so, when he was to undergo a gall-bladder operation himself, he used self-hypnosis as the only form of anaesthesia. The surgery was performed without complications or pain.

What evidence is there that hypnotherapy works?

As we learnt earlier, the practice of hypnosis is considerably older than academic research and older than any other modern medical practice. Hence, since the very early days of psychology, hypnosis has been subject to analysis and experiment. Thousands of books and articles have been published on the effects of hypnosis, containing references to research projects and case studies, which confirm the characteristics of hypnotic trance and its therapeutic benefits.

To pick just a few recent examples:

The **British Medical Journal** (BMJ) published a 'Clinical Review' of hypnosis and relaxation therapies (Vickers & Zolman, 1997) in which an overview of current medical research on hypnosis confirms its effectiveness in alleviating pain and treating various medical conditions.

In a recent review of eighteen studies on the effectiveness of hypnosis for pain management[2], the overall result was that most patients treated with hypnosis have moderate to significantly better surgical outcomes, including reports of less pain, use of fewer pain medications, and faster recovery. For example, medical hypnosis for orthopaedic hand surgery, which is typically very painful, showed benefits that included significantly less post-surgery pain and anxiety, and fewer complications.

A year 2000 review of published articles in the field of hypnosis concluded that "the research to date generally substantiates the claim that hypnotic procedures can ameliorate many psychological and medical conditions."[3]

Ginandes and Daniel Rosenthal, professor of radiology at the Harvard Medical School, published a report on their study of hypnosis to speed up the mending of broken bones. They recruited twelve people with broken ankles who did not require surgery and who received the usual treatment at Massachusetts General Hospital in Boston. In addition, Ginandes hypnotised half of them once a week for twelve weeks, while the other half received only normal treatment. The same doctor applied the casts and other care, and the same radiologists took regular X-rays to monitor how well they healed. A radiologist who evaluated the X-rays did not know which patients had undergone hypnosis.

The result stood out like a sore ankle. Those who were hypnotised healed faster than those who were not. Six weeks after the fracture, those in the hypnosis group showed the equivalent of eight-and-a-half weeks of healing.

Research on the use of hypnosis in obstetrics and maternity care

Hypnosis: practical applications and theoretical considerations in normal labour.
Jenkins, M. W. and Pritchard, M. H. Br J of Obstetrics and Gynaecology 1993 Mar; 100 (3): 221–6; Wales.

Two statistically significant findings include a *reduction in the length of active labour* (first-time mothers using hypnosis had 6.4 hours; the control group had 9.3 hours, p<0.0001); first-time mothers had a significantly *reduced incidence of pain medication use* (96% in the control group had nitrous oxide and/or Demerol vs. 74% in the hypnosis group, p<0.001).

Improved obstetric outcomes using hypnotic analgesia and skill mastery combined with childbirth education.

Harmon, Hynan and Tyre. J Consult Clin Psychol 1990 Oct; 58(5): 525–30; Milwaukee.
This randomised control trial reported **shorter labours, less medication use** and **less reported pain, higher APGAR scores**, more frequent **spontaneous deliveries** and reduced incidence of **postpartum depression**.

Hypnosis for Childbirth· prenatal education and labour outcome.
Shawn Gallagher, unpublished, October 2000; Toronto.

This retrospective survey for 31 low-risk first-time mothers notes average active labour of 3.75 hours (vs. 12 hours for the general population), an epidural rate of 16% (vs. 40–90% in Toronto and outlying areas), a Caesarian-section rate of 6.5% (vs. 20.1–36% in Toronto and outlying areas), reduced maternal pain perception, reduced intervention and a higher incidence of planned home births delivering at home (92%).

---

[1] Milton Erickson, "An Experimental Investigation of the Possible Anti-Social Use of Hypnosis", 1939, bc. cit.

[2] Montgomery, G. H., DuHamel, K. N. and Redd, W. N., 2000, "A meta-analysis of hypnotic analgesia: How effective is hypnosis?", *International Journal of Clinical and Experimental Hypnosis*, 48, 138–153.

[3] Montgomery, G. H., David, D., Winkel, G., Silverstein, J. H. and Bovbjerg, D. H. "The effectiveness of adjunctive hypnosis with surgical patients: A meta-analysis", *Anesthesia and Analgesia*, 94, 1639–1645.

Glossary for birth physiology

If you are unsure about any of the terminology, here is a guide to the different parts of your body involved with giving birth.

The pelvis

This is the cradle which supports all the reproductive organs and the bladder, intestines and rectum. It is the cradle that will support and protect the baby. It is a strong, bony ring which supports the weight of the body through the spinal column and then distributes the weight through the legs. The shape, flexibility and structure of the pelvis enables babies to be born.

The pelvis is made up of four bones – two hip bones, the sacrum, and the tail bone or coccyx. The hip bones are made up of three separate bones, which fuse over time into one solid plate. The sacrum lies between the two hip bones and is made up of fused vertebrae. The tail bone is the lower end of these fused bones; however, the tail bone can move and does so during birth to allow the baby to move down the birth canal. The bones and joints are held together by ligaments which become more flexible during pregnancy and birth, so that there is a degree of flexibility again to help the baby to be born. This is due to the hormones progesterone and relaxin. These ligaments are very strong and give extra reinforcing strength to the pelvis, especially during pregnancy.

For the vast majority of women, their body will not grow a baby that is too big to pass through their pelvis. Problems only really occur due to injury, disease, malnutrition or heredity.

The womb

The womb is a pear-shaped set of hollow muscles which nestles in the pelvic girdle.

It has three main areas:
- The fundus, which is the layer of muscle at the top of the womb.
- The body, which is the main chamber where the baby will grow.
- The cervix – a narrow canal of circular muscles with an opening at the bottom to let sperm in and to let the baby out.

The womb is made of very powerful muscles in three layers – the outer layer of muscle fibres are arranged long ways, the middle layer is made up of interlacing muscle fibres and blood vessels, and the inner layer are circular muscles. The outer longitudinal muscles are soft and supple and draw back the inner circular muscles at the neck of the womb – just like pulling a polo-neck jumper over your head! Thus the muscles of the womb work in harmony to open the cervix and then push the baby out of the woman's body.

The uterus

The uterus is the more commonly used term given to the womb once the baby has started growing. The uterus is the most amazing organ, with an enormous potential and capacity for growth and immense power.

During pregnancy, the uterus grows from the size of a small pear to the size of a big watermelon. The weight goes from about 60 grams up to a kilo. In the beginning, it is an almost solid structure; by the end, it has thinned out to become like a large inflated balloon, yet it is strong enough to push out a ten-pound baby or more, plus a large placenta.

In a pregnant woman, it is the largest bag of muscles in her body, and so when it flexes you can really feel it as a powerful sensation, similar to Jane Fonda's "the burn". But always remember that the muscles of the uterus will work for you no matter what you do. Even if a woman were unconscious or in a coma, the muscles of the uterus would birth her baby.

The cervix

This is not actually a separate structure, as it is simply the end of the uterus. However, people talk so much of the cervix that it deserves its own section. During pregnancy, the cervix feels a bit like a gristly nose – quite long and circular – and stays firmly closed with a mucus plug in the opening to prevent any infection going into the uterus. This plug will come out as the cervix begins to soften in the days before labour begins. In the build-up to and during labour, the cervix will thin out, soften and begin to move up into the uterus. Once labour begins, the cervix will then begin to open.

The cervix is the part of the woman's body which is commonly measured to ascertain how far along she is in labour. There is a common belief that a cervix will dilate one centimetre per hour – this is highly inaccurate. All cervixes perform in their own way and there is no real set pattern as to how fast or slow a cervix will open. As the long muscles of the uterus reach down, they gradually pull back the circular muscles to allow them to open. This basically incorporates the cervix into the body of the uterus.

However, the circular muscles have to soften and move into the right position, and this can take many hours of contractions. Often the hardest part is getting the cervix to soften (ripen) and open the first 2–3 cm. During this time, women are not deemed to be in "active labour". Once those first few centimetres have been reached, the cervix can dilate quite quickly or can carry on at a slower pace.

A cervix can be felt quite near the entrance of the vagina, and the degree of opening can be assessed by a midwife (vaginal examination). She will gently insert two fingers into the vagina and, depending on the opening of the cervix, she will judge how far apart her fingers are, and thus how many centimetres open the cervix is.

Once the cervix is about 10 cm, it is large enough for the baby to pass through. As the cervix retracts up into the uterus, the neck of the uterus becomes thicker and longer, acting like a piston to push out the baby.

The birth canal

The canal or passage from the neck of the womb to the outside wall is made up of multi-folded skin. This allows for the canal to open to many times its normal size. There are also two small lubricating glands on either side, which help to lubricate the canal both during love-making and during childbirth, making the passage extra slippery.

The canal is about 7.5 cm long at the front and about 10 cm long at the back. The area is incredibly rich in very tiny blood vessels, so that, even if there is damage or a tear, the blood loss will be minimal, as the vessels are so small.

Once the cervix is open, the ridges in the vagina – normally there to create pleasure during love-making – disappear and become excessively lubricated.

There is a direct correlation of the muscles of the mouth with the muscles of the birth canal. It is therefore very important that a birthing mother keep her mouth, jaw and neck loose and relaxed. A great way to do this is to do "horse breathing" – or blowing air rapidly though closed lips. This is a great exercise, as it is often easier for a woman to focus on relaxing her mouth and jaw than it is to relax her perineum. Other ways would be to use singing, humming or low-pitched moaning as a great way to relax the muscles of the neck and throat.

The pelvic floor

The pelvic floor is a hammock-like set of muscles, ligaments and connective tissue. It is a very strong group of muscles and again supports the inner organs as well as the growing baby. The muscles help the peristaltic motion of the sphincter muscles of the anus, urethra and cervix. As these muscles support the bladder and urethra, any weakness of the muscles can lead to the sphincters not being as efficient as they can be, which can lead to incontinence, especially when sneezing, laughing or coughing.

During childbirth, these muscles are relaxed and opened to a great extent, so if the muscle tone is not strong, there is an increased chance of the muscles becoming weaker after the baby is born. It is therefore important for women to do pelvic-floor exercises throughout pregnancy and beyond.

The perineum

The perineum is a diamond-shaped set of muscles just under the pelvic floor, between the vagina and anus. Again, these muscles are folded and thick so that they have the ability to stretch to a size that would allow the baby's head and body to be born. However, it is useful for a mother to massage the perineum regularly in the later stages of pregnancy to increase the suppleness of the muscle tissue.

In more traditional societies, women had far stronger pelvic floors and perineal muscles, as much of their time was spent walking and squatting, both of which would strengthen the muscles. In modern society, women spend far too much time sitting, which leads to the muscles weakening.

The placenta

When the placenta comes out of the body, it is a large, reddish-blue, liver-like organ with an amazing network of blood vessels on one side, which resemble a tree in winter. A placenta can be 15–20 cm in diameter and about 3 cm thick. It is the lifeline for the baby and acts as the kidneys, liver, lungs and intestines.

All the baby's blood and nutrition passes through the placenta, which is made up of tissue from both the mother and the baby. Although the mother and baby's blood does not actually mix, the vessels are so close that oxygen and nutrients pass through the arteries from the mother's blood into the baby's blood, and the carbon dioxide and waste products transfer from the baby's into the mother's blood.

The umbilical cord

The cord connects the placenta to the baby – it is the lifeline between the mother and the baby. It is made up of a vein and two arteries, which are covered in a rubbery, whitish-grey substance. The cord varies in length, but is usually about 2 cm thick and about 50 cm long, or long enough for the baby to lie by the mother's breast after the birth without stretching the cord.

It has become common for the umbilical cord to be cut after the baby is born. This is done mainly for convenience, so that the mother can move away from the baby; however, traditionally, the cord would not be cut and would be left attached to the baby and placenta until it naturally dropped off about three days after the birth (known as a lotus birth).

If the cord is to be cut, it is important to leave the cord until it has stopped pulsating. That way, the baby is benefiting from getting oxygen from breathing whilst still getting oxygenated blood through the cord. Once it has stopped pulsating, there is no more movement between the placenta and the baby, and it is safe to clamp and then cut the cord.

Amniotic fluid

In the womb, the baby is surrounded by salty fluid called amniotic fluid. It acts as a protector and shock absorber for the baby, helps the baby maintain its temperature, and allows the baby to move freely and easily in the womb. The body is continually making amniotic fluid, replenishing the fluid every 3–4 hours. In the womb, the baby will drink-in the amniotic fluid and will pee into the water (or fluid), which is then passed through the mother's system and out in her urine. This continuous production of amniotic fluid makes it even more important that a pregnant woman drink plenty of liquid.

When the baby is ready to be born, there is between a litre and a litre and a half around the baby. The fluid is held in by a membrane around the baby. As the baby is getting ready to be born, the pressure of the baby's head may lead to the membrane releasing and letting some of the amniotic fluid out. This is known as "the waters breaking" or "membranes rupturing".

The baby's head

For many women, one of the greatest fears is how they are going to pass a baby's head through an opening which is essentially nowhere near that size. As you will have read, many things occur during childbirth to help this process; however, it is useful to understand a little about the structure of the baby's head.

Generally, the head is the largest and least-compressible part of the baby's body. The skull is made up of three sections – the top of the head, the face, and the base of the skull. The second two are fused and so do not move. However, the top of the skull is made up of several bones, which are connected by flexible membranes. Where these bones are held together, there are soft spots on the baby's skull – called fontanels. This means that those bones actually move and slide over each other, so the skull gets moulded during the birth, especially as the baby moves down the birth canal. The contents of the baby's skull do not get compressed, just moved around, so the skull gets longer.

Natal Hypnotherapy tracks and courses

Voted 'Pregnancy Product of the Year' by *Practical Parenting* magazine

The Natal Hypnotherapy range of tracks has been developed to enhance your conception, pregnancy and birth experience by using your natural skills and inner resources. By listening to the tracks, you learn a combination of self-hypnosis techniques, deep relaxation and guided visualisation to help you overcome fears, create a state of calm and relaxation, maintain your health, increase bonding with your baby, and maximise your body's potential.

By rehearsing the way you would like things to be – for example, a comfortable, natural birth – over and over again in your mind, it becomes more and more familiar to you, and so effectively you remove the fear of the unknown.

"One of the main keys to a successful labour is being calm, relaxed and feeling in control. From my observations, hypnotherapy certainly helps to promote relaxation.

Some of our clients who have used hypnosis antenatally have reported that they have been able to 'self-hypnotise' during labour, making it an easier and enjoyable experience. One client was so relaxed after using the track that it hardly seemed as though she was labouring."

Laura Abbott, Midwife

The current range of tracks includes:

- The IVF Companion
- Prepare to Conceive
- Overcome Morning Sickness
- Letting go of fear
- Easy to sleep
- Pregnancy Relaxation
- Pregnancy Relaxation (twins)
- Hospital Birth Preparation
- Hospital Birth preparation (twins)
- Home Birth Preparation

- Home Birth Preparation (twins)
- Prepare for a Caesarean
- Prepare for a Caesarean (twins)
- VBAC Preparation
- The Labour Companion
- Fast Postnatal Recovery
- Fast Postnatal Recovery (twins)
- Breastfeeding Companion

Whatever stage you're at, Natal Hypnotherapy can help you.

Pre - Conception	0 - 32 weeks	32 - 40+ weeks	Birth	Postnatal
Prepare to Conceive	Pregnancy Relaxation	Birth Preparation	Relaxing Birth Music	Fast Postnatal Recovery
IVF Companion	Overcoming Morning Sickness		Labour Companion	Breastfeeding Companion

4 CD Programme includes:

Options:
Hospital/Birth Centre
Home
VBAC
Twins
Caesarean
Caesarean Twins

To understand how effective the Natal Hypnotherapy methos have been for mothers, every mother who buys a track from the www.natalhypnotherapy.co.uk website is sent a postnatal questionnaire six weeks after their baby is due.

The following statistics are based on feedback from 769 mothers.

97% of mothers would recommend Natal Hypnotherapy to others

90% said they had **benefited from** using the tracks

83.6% felt they were very or extremely **relaxed** going into the birth

77.4% felt they were relaxed or very **relaxed during the birth**

80% felt they **overcame fear** and anxiety leading up to the birth

80% felt able to manage or **deal with** the level of **pain** during birth

88% went into the birth with a strong **belief in their body's** ability to give birth

The Caesarean rate is 15% compared to the UK national rate of 24%

"All your tracks helped me so much. I was someone who was really scared, but felt so relaxed and in control in my pregnancy and the birth. I used the postnatal recovery at the hospital, which made me feel calm, in control and confident, and I am sure my daughter is so good because I am so calm and confident. Thank you so much!" **Fiona Whittaker**

"I feel that I had a very positive birth experience and real empowerment by that. I definitely feel that the hypnotherapy CDs helped us to achieve this and that they helped to diminish some of the fear and anxiety, and therefore pain, of the experience." **Jennie Shales**

"I always looked forward to the birth, and I believe that was down to NH. I can't tell enough mums about how good the experience was, and without any pain relief! I felt everything and it was fantastic – THANK YOU!!!" **Donna Lynch**

Natal Hypnotherapy course (in person and online)

"This course reaches the parts that other antenatal courses do not reach!"

Natal Hypnotherapy course has been run in the UK since 2003 and has helped support thousands of couples through their pregnancy and birth journey.

Reading a book or listening to a track can help in many ways; however, there is no real substitute for getting together with an experienced person in order to learn and practise hands-on tools and techniques.

The courses are fun, inspiring, and practical, and truly help couples feel as if they are in charge of their birth preparation. They teach couples a wide range of practical tools and techniques to overcome their fears and to help them feel more confident, trusting and in control.

Courses are geared very much at both the mother and her birth partner, as we believe that if both of you are working as a team, and both feel relaxed and confident, then you have the best-possible chance of having a wonderful and positive birth experience. The courses cover:

1. Natural pain relief for birth

- Natural ways to reduce pain in childbirth
- Self-hypnosis skills to overcome fear and increase your confidence and trust in your ability to give birth
- Effective breathing and deep-relaxation techniques
- How fear or anxiety can have a negative impact on your body during the birth, and learning how to reduce it
- Ways your birth partner can help you achieve a deeply relaxed state

2. Practical birth preparation

- Practical techniques to help you stay calm and relaxed during the birth, including massage, using a birth ball, and birthing positions
- How your body works best during labour and what you can do to help it
- Practical tools and techniques for your partner to keep you calm and relaxed and to ease discomfort during the birth
- How your emotions change during the labour, and signs to look for

"I just wanted to say a huge thank you for your fantastic course. I finally gave birth ten days late and have just had the most amazing experience of my life!

My midwife kept commenting that she'd never seen anyone so relaxed! I felt so in control, and totally able to breathe through the contractions. The most amazing part was the birth itself. It went exactly as I had dreamed and hoped it would: just breathing the baby through the birth canal, then one push for the head, one for the body.

I really appreciate everything you taught us: to experience such a wonderful birth after such a terrible one last time was just fantastic. I've found it so easy to adjust and recover. Thank you so much for teaching me your amazing skills – I'd recommend the course to anyone!"

Cathy and Steve Smith

"Even though we had a few challenges during the birth, we were both really happy with the whole experience under the circumstances and, thanks to you, felt informed and able to ask for things to be done the way we wanted. I am convinced that the techniques I learnt with you enabled me to cope in an environment that felt very alien and not at all relaxing. I religiously listened to your CD every day after the course and I really did feel in control, which is amazing under the circumstances."

Kevin and Estelle

"Thanks for a great two days. It was really useful for me to understand about the phases of birth and how to deal with the medical team, and to be given an important role in the whole process. I particularly enjoyed the hypnosis sessions and felt very comfortable asking any questions and talking about my fears."

Michael, London

Courses are held throughout the UK. To find a practitioner near you go to www.natalhypnotherapy.co.uk

The online course is available 24 /7 and is in a modular format so you can access the course around your own schedule from the comfort of your own home. http://best.hypnobirthingclass.online/courses/hypnobirthing

Other ways to make your pregnancy and birth comfortable and enjoyable

Acupuncture

Acupuncture has been around for over five-thousand years. It is based on the belief that an internal force of energy runs through the body. It brings relief of pain which may be unresponsive to conventional therapy or painkillers. It brings with it a feeling of relaxation after the therapy. It helps to re balance the body's own energy

Use in pregnancy:
Acupuncture is most widely used to correct foetal malposition, e.g. babies lying in a breech position.

Acupuncture can also help with metabolic problems, nausea, heartburn, headache (migraine), anxiety and insomnia. Piles, varicose veins and fluid retention also respond well to treatment.

Use in labour:
It can help to induce labour and ease pain. Many studies show that women receiving acupuncture report a sense of well-being and calm and of being in control of their own labour and delivery.

Postnatal:
It can help with heavy blood loss, lactation problems and postnatal depression.

What to expect:
Acupuncture is virtually painless. Fine, sterile needles are used and only penetrate the superficial layers of the skin.

Your therapist may use a variety of techniques to stimulate acupuncture points, such as finger pressure, massage, electricity (TENS machine) and heat (moxa).

Your therapist may also make dietary recommendations to help with the demands of nourishing the foetus and providing milk after the birth.

Rescue Remedy

Rescue Remedy is a Bach flower remedy, which can be very beneficial for use in birthing. You can buy it in most pharmacies. It comes in the form of a tincture, in a small bottle with a dropper, and is made from several flower essences. It is very calming and relaxing. Put several drops in your drinking water throughout labour. You can also put a few drops directly into your mouth (or your partner's!) if you feel faint, tense, stressed or afraid at any time.

Rescue Remedy is very helpful during transition and can also be used just before any medical intervention.

Chiropractor

What it is:
Chiropractic is a straightforward method of adjusting the bones of your body to relieve pain and restore movement. Chiropractors believe that any disturbance of the musculo-skeletal system will not only cause local pain, but also interfere with the body's other main components.

Use in pregnancy/labour:
The gentle nature of chiropractic makes it especially suitable during pregnancy. The whole-body approach can enhance the health and well-being of both mother and baby. Misalignments of the spine caused by pregnancy can change your posture and press on nerves, which in turn causes not only back pain but pain that can affect the whole body. Treatment aims to realign the body's structure.

What to expect:
On your first visit, you will be asked for a full history of your health and well-being. Your chiropractor will then examine the joints in your body using their hands and will make appropriate adjustments. You can start receiving treatments after the first three months of pregnancy.

Reflexology

What it is:
Reflexology aims to treat the whole body through the feet. There are specific areas which represent all parts of the body. Similar reflexes are also found on the hand. Reflexologists believe that where there is an imbalance in the body, small crystals form in the corresponding part of the feet. Massaging the feet can help to break up the crystals, thus allowing the body's internal energy to circulate freely.

Use in pregnancy:
Reflexology is very relaxing and can help with general anxiety and well-being as well as helping specific conditions, such as early-morning sickness, constipation and migraines.

Use in labour:
Can help as a natural form of induction to bring on labour. During labour, massaging certain points will help with relaxation and the stimulation of oxytocin (birthing hormones), and so help with pain relief.

Osteopathy

What it is:
Osteopathy is now one of the most widely practised complementary therapies in the West. Osteopaths believe that the musculo-skeletal system plays a vital part in the health of the body and that any misalignment can cause a reduction in circulation, leading to various ailments.

Use in pregnancy:
Osteopathy can be helpful to relieve joint and muscular problems, including sciatica, head-aches, back and neck pain.

What to expect:
As osteopathy is a "holistic" treatment, your therapist will firstly take your full medical history, before examining your posture and your spine. This will be followed by skilful realignment or release of the vertebrae and joints. Often there is an accompanying "click".

Cranial osteopathy can also help with postnatal depression and with your child after they have been born, particularly unsettled, colicky babies.

Yoga

What it is:
Yoga is a therapy recognised in helping stress, improving joint and muscle suppleness, and generally improving overall health and well-being.

Use in pregnancy:
The breathing and body awareness help you stay connected to your changing body. With so many changes taking place, it is a wonderful time to slow down and appreciate your baby and the amazing ability of your body. The gentle moving therapy works well in pregnancy, especially

for problems with backache and posture. Regular yoga can also help increase the suppleness of the pelvic floor, thereby reducing the risk of damage during labour.

Use in labour:
Antenatal yoga classes teach effective breathing techniques for the birth. Yoga teaches you to trust your body, to focus and to work with your body through the birth. Yoga also increases the suppleness in your pelvic-floor muscles, which may make your labour easier, and helps these muscles recover quickly after birth.

Hiring a doula

What is a doula?
A doula is a trained birth companion who will support the parents during pregnancy and throughout the birth. A doula believes in "mothering the mother", thus enabling a woman to have the most satisfying and positive experience.

What does a doula do?
A doula will listen, encourage and support both parents in their birth choices. She will be on hand to answer questions and offer advice and reassurance. She will be with the mother before, during and after the birth, offering emotional and physical support. A doula does not replace a midwife and does not have medical training.

How can a doula help?
Research has shown that a mother who is attended by a trusted, loving companion throughout her labour is far more likely to have a normal birth. If a mother feels loved and supported throughout the birth, she will be more relaxed, calmer, and more confident, which in turn will empower her to have a better birth experience.

Your personal notes

These pages are a place to write your own notes, affirmations, suggestions, metaphors, etc.

Letting go

Write down any particular metaphors or methods that you feel would help you release and let go of any fears. Use these at any time during your pregnancy and birth, when fears or concerns occupy your mind. This is especially useful during the birth to help you acknowledge, accept and then let go.

_____

_____

_____

_____

_____

_____

_____

_____

_____

_____

_____

_____

_____

_____

_____

_____

_____

_____

_____

_____

_____

_____

_____

_____

Affirmations

Write down any particular affirmations that will help you feel confident, inspired and motivated. You can write these on cards and place them around your home or put them in a bowl on the kitchen table. You can then pick one up at random and read it for inspiration or if you are feeling a little down or concerned.

_____

_____

_____

_____

_____

_____

_____

_____

_____

_____

_____

_____

_____

_____

_____

_____

_____

_____

_____

_____

_____

_____

_____

_____

_____

Triggers

Triggers work best when they are personal and have meaning to you. A trigger can be anything from a few words, such as '3, 2, 1, relax', to a feeling, such as a hand on your shoulder, or an image, for example a special photograph.

Use this page to write down a few triggers that you or your birth partner can use during the labour, and the response that you would like each one to bring about, for example relaxation, calm, deep breathing, trust, and so on.

Auditory - 3. 2. 1 Relax

Visual - Little Bubs teddy

My comfort measures

Use this to write down any tools or techniques that you and your birth partner can use during the birth itself. This may include the visualisations and metaphors that you include in your birth script as well as the physical comfort measures from step 5.

Visualisation
~ Chamonix / Being in the Mountains / Himalayas

~ Christmas ~ sound of carols, taste of mince pies, twinkling lights, smell of tree.

~ Beach ~ Galapagos, sea turtles

Birth partner's notes

Use this page to note down all the things you can do to support and help during the birth, including comfort measures, metaphors, BRAINs, things to remember, and so on.

_____
_____
_____
_____
_____
_____
_____
_____
_____
_____
_____
_____
_____
_____
_____
_____
_____
_____
_____
_____
_____
_____
_____
_____
_____
_____
_____
_____
_____
_____
_____

Your birth mind map

Use this space to create your birth mind map – remember to focus on what you want and on the emotional, as well as the physical, journey of birth.

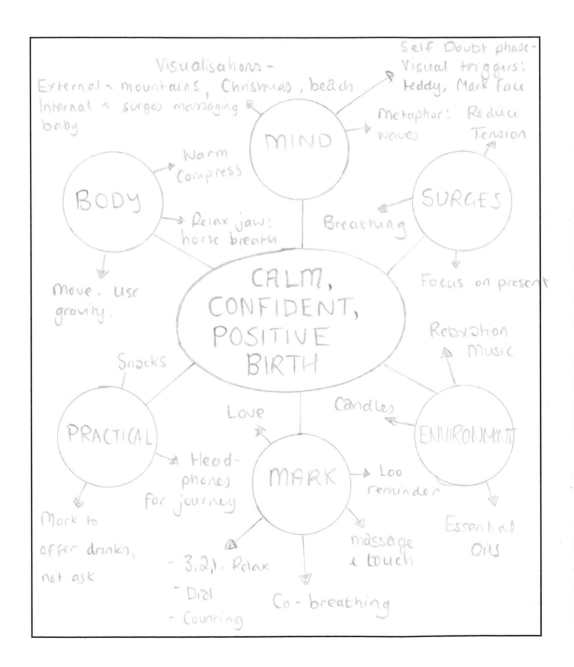

Your birth script

This is where you can bring together everything that you have learnt. Once you have read this book, take some time out to really think about the key things you want to feel and experience during your birth. Imagine that you have a crystal ball and that you can see into the future to see how your birth unfolds.

Write it from an "internal" perspective – that is, what you are feeling rather than where you are, what time it is, the people around you, etc. Include your triggers, e.g. "every time I feel my partner stroke my arm, I become more and more relaxed and calm". Use metaphors such as "with each contraction, my body feels as if it is a floppy rag doll". That way, your partner need simply say the words "floppy rag doll" and your subconscious will recall the meaning.

This is not a birth plan – it is simply a way to give your subconscious an image of what you expect and hope will happen, as well as how you would like to respond to the changes in your body that are definitely going to happen.

_____
_____
_____
_____
_____
_____
_____
_____
_____
_____
_____
_____
_____
_____
_____
_____
_____
_____

Notes

_____
_____
_____
_____
_____
_____
_____
_____
_____
_____
_____
_____
_____
_____
_____
_____
_____
_____
_____
_____
_____
_____
_____
_____
_____
_____
_____
_____
_____
_____
_____

Index